Integration of Clinical and Financial Information Systems

Contributors

Carolyn Anderson-Stewart   Kathleen T. Lucke

Gerald E. Bisbee, Jr.   Marilyn P. Plomann

Barbara J. Brown   Linda J. Porter-Stubbs

Douglas A. Conrad   Marilyn L. Price

Truman H. Esmond, Jr.   Austin Ross

Anna Ferguson   David B. Starkweather

Joseph S. Gonnella   Vandan Trivedi

Mary Alice Krill   Carter Zeleznik

Integration
of Clinical
and Financial
Information Systems

Edited by

Barbara J. Brown, R.N., Ed.D., F.A.A.N
Assistant Administrator
Virginia Mason Medical Center
Seattle, Washington

Austin Ross, M.P.H., F.A.C.H.A.
Executive Vice President
Virginia Mason Medical Center
Seattle, Washington

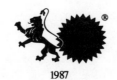

AN ASPEN PUBLICATION®
Aspen Publishers, Inc.

1987

Rockville, Maryland
Royal Tunbridge Wells

Library of Congress Cataloging in Publication Data

Integration of clinical and financial information systems.

Based on the Symposium on Contemporary Issues in Health Care, held Nov. 11-12, 1983, in Seattle, Wash., and sponsored by the Virginia Mason Medical Foundation and the Hospital Research and Educational Trust.

"An Aspen publication."
Includes bibliographies and index.
1. Information storage and retrieval systems—Hospitals—Congresses. 2. Hospitals—Finance—Data processing—Congresses. 3. Hospital records—Data processing—Congresses. 4. Diagnosis related groups—Data processing—Congresses. 5. Hospitals—Prospective payment—Data processing—Congresses. I. Brown, Barbara J. II. Ross, Austin. III. Symposium on Contemporary Issues in Health Care (1983: Seattle, Wash.) IV. Virginia Mason Medical Foundation. V. Hospital Research and Educational Trust. [DNLM: 1. Economics, Hospital—congresses. 2. Hospital Administration—congresses. 3. Information Systems—congresses. WX 157 I61 1983]
RA971.6.I58   1986   362.1'1'068   86-22151
ISBN: 0-87189-391-6

Editorial Services: Carolyn Ormes

Library of Congress Catalog Card Number: 86-22151
ISBN: 0-87189-391-6

Printed in the United States of America

1 2 3 4 5

Table of Contents

Foreword

As is stated repeatedly, the health delivery system is in a period of rapid change. In the mid-1980s and into the foreseeable future, policy and operating decisions are being driven by external competitive economic and regulatory factors. The dramatic reduction in hospital patients' length of stay, stimulated by Medicare's major modifications in payment mechanisms to hospitals in 1984, proved to be the latest weapon in the continuing battle to contain costs. Of special interest to medical economists was the fact that the implementation of the diagnosis related groups (DRGs), while applicable initially to Medicare patients, somehow worked also to reduce the length of stay for non-Medicare patients.

Physicians did not differentiate between Medicare and non-Medicare patients. They apparently did not treat patients differently, based on the payment method. This should not have come as any great surprise, particularly since the physicians were not at economic risk for the patients' care.

However, the introduction of capped payments based on diagnosis placed hospitals in the interesting position of having to consider how to influence the allocation of their resources to avoid losses. From the hospitals' viewpoint, it was fortunate that the implementation strategy for DRGs provided payment levels that left some room for error and, equally important, time for the system to adjust.

It is important to remember that although there had been some experimentation with capped payments, the New Jersey prospective payment method as the pilot model for DRGs being the most notable example, there was relatively little experience as to how such systems could be applied on a national basis. The grand experiment was implemented successfully and proved to be a turning point by demonstrating that costs could be contained if providers could be made to bear some direct risk and responsibility for these expenditures.

As hospital occupancy dropped, another force entered the picture—competition. Hospitals began to look for ways to strengthen their financial base. One way to do this was to increase market share. In a relatively static marketplace, this meant attracting patients from someone else. Competition, of course, took many forms. Hospitals began to examine, with much greater vigor, market research reports that identified patient demographics. New attention was placed on examining alternatives to hospitalization as a means of strengthening market share. Were there ways to use the hospitals' capital base to create joint venture patient service arrangements with physicians, group practices, skilled nursing facilities, home health care agencies, or other providers?

If the patient base was shifting to out-of-hospital service, then institutions had better accelerate their involvement through diversification or suffer the consequences.

In addition to competition, public and business concern about health care costs generated more fuel in the debate on the virtues of hospital rate regulation. While some state legislatures forged ahead to expand rate regulation, other states embraced the concept of free enterprise economics and began to eliminate regulations, including the certificate-of-need statutes. Some economists also observed that several of the most regulated states had among the highest per diem hospital costs in the nation.

Monitors of change noted with considerable interest the growth of alternative delivery systems. Wall Street discovered health maintenance organizations (HMOs). Preferred provider organizations (PPOs) began to flourish. These models were designed to respond to the driving force to achieve cost containment by putting providers at risk. This was the point at which business and industry began to appreciate how runaway health care costs could affect their profit bottom line immediately and profoundly.

Insurance companies, picking up on the new environment and recognizing the vulnerability of hospitals to declining occupancy, discovered that facilities would discount prices in order to take advantage of volume. Once hospitals engaged in discounting prices charged to their preferred customers, they learned how to provide services more inexpensively.

The combined forces of regulation and competition required new management techniques to track consumption of resources within the hospitals. This in turn led to the conclusion that there had to be improvements in the organizations' ability to link and integrate clinical and financial information. It also was not just the internal tracking systems that became of paramount importance, but the tracking of expenditures of capital used to expand services in the expectation of accessing new revenue sources.

The capital shortfall, or at least the fear of a capital shortfall, accelerated the speed of change. Some larger hospitals feared that over time they no longer would be able to access capital in sufficient quantity. They turned to consideration of alternatives, one of which was to sell out to a larger corporation.

Other issues surfaced as the financial base shifted:

- Would rural hospitals survive?
- Would suburban hospitals, with their lower cost base, be able to outbid downtown urban institutions for patients, thereby jeopardizing the urban facilities' ability to continue their support of medical education, charity care, new technology, or research?
- Would purchasers of care recognize the importance of supporting some of these needs, or would they take a shortcut approach to reduce health care expenditures?

All of these factors, taken in turn, could be dealt with in a somewhat predictable fashion. But the cumulative impact of the magnitude of the new measures on an industry known for its consistency and predictability led to an unprecedented speed of change.

This book addresses the importance and impact of tracking the consumption of hospital services as the means through which institutions and their staffs can contain costs, share risks, and maintain the health system's financial viability and quality. History is in the making and the speed of change will continue to accelerate. It is an exciting era for hospitals, their managements, boards, and staffs—and for the purchasers of health care.

Austin Ross

Preface

The design of an integrated clinical and financial data base is viewed by many as an extremely powerful tool of the 1980s to contain health care costs and to assure optimal use of medical resources. With 10 percent of the gross national product being allocated to health care costs, the federal government initiated a revolutionary method of reimbursing for Medicare patients that involves the establishment of a flat reimbursement rate to hospitals based on the diagnosis or condition being treated. This effectively placed a cap on reimbursement and provided targets for repayment for each institution. If the cost of serving a patient exceeds the generally established limits, hospitals are forced to absorb the loss; conversely, if hospitals can provide services at less than established rates, then they will participate in some incentive returns. The success of this type of payment system depends to a substantial degree on the quality and application of clinical and financial data systems.

These data systems, which establish profiles for institutions, also are providing information to purchasers of health services concerning trends and patterns in the costs of care. There is much controversy about the effectiveness of this type of payment system and its effects on the cost and quality of care. A comprehensive exploration of clinical and financial data systems that can be integrated effectively and can explain the systems' impact on the traditional service product is a significant contribution to the literature for health care executives.

This book contributes new information to aid in the design of significant health systems changes that already are well under way. It thoroughly reviews the issues, solidly forecasts future effects of clinical and financial data systems changes on the health care field, and identifies specific areas for future research.

On November 11-12, 1983, a Symposium on Contemporary Issues in Health Care took place in Seattle, Washington. This conference was funded in part through a grant from Citicorp Inc. (USA) of New York. As a result of the dialogue and the seeking of answers for difficult questions, this book came into being.

Barbara Brown

Acknowledgments

We are particularly indebted to Mr. Robert T. Jacobs, Vice President and Area Manager, Citicorp Inc., for his encouragement and involvement in the Symposium on Contemporary Issues in Health Care, as a result of which this book came to be written. Special acknowledgment and appreciation is given to all the participants in the symposium, six of whom contributed to chapters in this book:

Gerald E. Bisbee, Jr., Ph.D.
Barbara J. Brown, R.N., Ed.D., F.A.A.N.
Douglas A. Conrad, Ph.D.
Robert A. DeVries, M.B.A.
Truman H. Esmond, Jr., M.A.S.
L. Frederick Fenster, M.D.
Joseph S. Gonnella, M.D.
C. Reiley Kidd, M.D.
Mary Alice Krill, Ph.D.
Jack O. Lanier, Ph.D., F.A.C.H.A.
John W. Lewis, III, Ph.D.
Leo K. Lichtig, Ph.D.
Daniel Z. Louis, M.S.
Regina McPhillips, Ph.D.
John P. Mamana, M.D.
Donald R. Olson, M.H.A.
Lowell E. Palmquist, M.H.A.
Marilyn P. Plomann, M.S.M.
John Rasmussen, Ph.D.
J. Michael Rona, M.H.A.
Austin Ross, M.P.H., F.A.C.H.A.
Dale N. Schumacher, M.D.

David B. Starkweather, Ph.D.
John D. Thompson, M.H.A.
June Werner, R.N., M.N., M.S.N., C.N.A.A.

We also thank Donna Ohman, administrative secretary at Virginia Mason Hospital, Seattle, for her time, patience, and support in pooling the manuscripts and assisting in the final production of the manuscript.

Introduction

A Symposium on Contemporary Issues in Health Care: Integration of Clinical and Financial Data Systems

Austin Ross

The stimulus for studying the impact of data on health services delivery has a long history. Health service, as any other service or product, has costs associated with its creation and delivery. Its delivery is complicated because of the nature of the service. Several unique distinctions bear on how decisions are made by consumers of health services and how these services are paid for.

Patients, for example, have not always been in the best position to make decisions or choices of when or how care is to be received. A health crisis places decisions in the hands of others. The physicians determine, for the most part, the timing and the means of diagnosis and treatment. Decisions on which hospital to use have been based, not on relative prices, but on where the attending physicians had hospital privileges.

Generally, in the past, with the exception of a handful of closed system entities such as health maintenance organizations (HMOs), which functioned on a capitation system, patients and their physicians had a wide variety of choices of where to go for care. As the health system matured, the methods of payment began to influence these decisions. Medicare with its cost-reimbursement methodology certainly encouraged wider use by providing its beneficiaries with the insurance protection needed to assure access to care. The cost-reimbursement system also provided physicians, hospitals, nursing homes, and other institutions and professionals with the assurance that payments would be received for services rendered.

Over the years, Blue Cross, Blue Shield, and the insurance industry provided a wide variety of employer- or employee-paid health insurance programs. Since some of these were based on costs and some on prices, the payment levels varied according to the type of payer. Cost shifting became a way of life. As cost-based payers redefined expenditures, these reductions were recaptured by adding to the prices charged to insurance companies, which paid by price.

The important factor, however, was that under either a cost-based or a price-based system, there were few incentives to relate costs of the service to the rate of

utilization. It was with the emergence of systems that placed hospitals or other providers at risk for the quantity of care given that attention began to focus on
deficiencies of data collection and usage.

In fact, major institutions generally maintained separate systems for financial
and clinical data. There was no apparent need to merge these systems until it
became apparent that cost containment meant that the volume of services ultimately would be capped and the providers (in this case the hospitals) would be put
at financial risk.

The integration of clinical and financial data systems suddenly moved from
being almost exclusively the domain of health system economists and researchers
to being the domain of health executives, medical and nursing staffs, insurance
actuaries, and employers.

The chapters that follow take this one step further and not only focus on data
issues but also discuss the impact of data integration on the organization, the
professional staff, and the system as a whole.

This book results from a Seattle conference cosponsored by the Virginia Mason
Medical Foundation and the Hospital Research and Educational Trust of the
American Hospital Association. The Trust's interest stems from a number of its
studies, the most notable being a project to develop a planning, budgeting, and
clinical management system based on the integrated financial and clinical data
streams of the hospital. This project was funded by the W. J. Kellogg Foundation
and the Duke Endowment. Virginia Mason Medical Center's interest developed
through a grant from the Northwest Area Foundation to develop a case intensity
tool based on combining clinical and financial data.

The pioneering work of Riedel, followed by that of Thompson, Fetter, and
others on diagnosis related groups, and the substantial implementation efforts in
New Jersey, provided numerous clues to the new directions for payment mechanisms.

It was with this background in mind that representatives of Virginia Mason
contacted Gerald E. Bisbee, Jr., then president of the Educational and Research
Trust, to ascertain whether the Trust would be interested in cosponsoring a "think
tank" approach to examine in depth this topic of merging data systems. An
affirmative response from the Trust, coupled with a generous grant from Citicorp,
provided the means to carry the project forward.

It was determined early that the number of participants would be limited. Those
invited would bring a special level of expertise to the conference table. The group
would include some from the academic and research community, and others with
interest and knowledge in management, medicine, nursing, medical records, and,
of course, data processing.

The conference was short—a Friday noon through Saturday afternoon—but the
pace and level of expectations were high. Primary participants were asked to
submit manuscripts a month in advance. These in turn were distributed to partici-

pants several days before the meeting and all were asked to review the material, including conference objectives. Complete curricula vitae on all participants were distributed and considerable care was taken to set the stage properly. The expertise of the group demanded that the time and efforts be focused for maximum return.

From the beginning of planning for the conference, efforts were directed at producing a product that would be usable. This book, of course, meets that objective. Of considerable value to the Virginia Mason organization was that the gathering in Seattle of some of the nation's experts in data collection and usage, and on a topic of such import, provided considerable impetus to the organization's push for programs involving the merging of such data. The importance of this venture should not be minimized.

The outcome of the conference affected the Virginia Mason Medical Center in a number of ways. The medical staff, for example, accessing conference information in a timely fashion, was in a better position to prepare for DRGs. Management subsequently, and ahead of time, devoted more resources to the difficult task of refining data base banks.

Virginia Mason is involved in a consortium almost two decades old, consisting of 13 community and rural hospitals in southwest Washington. These hospitals, through accessing medical records and other disciplines, were better prepared for the implementation of the prospective payment system.

Since one of the goals of the conference was to identify research topics for further study, both the Trust and Virginia Mason benefited, as it was hoped all participants did through the process of the networking of vital information.

The objectives of the conference can be summarized as follows:

1. to collect and disseminate information on the necessity of integrating clinical and financial information
2. to conduct a conference capable of producing a synergistic impact on the participants in order to reinforce further long-range work in data system development
3. to create (at Virginia Mason) a greater appreciation of the need to increase its investment in data and control systems in order to prepare for the future.

It is the editors' conviction that this conference met its objectives. But there was one additional hidden agenda item that should be mentioned. It is this author's conviction that it is crucial for the academic and the practice communities to meet to discuss topics of import. It is not easy to assemble a group of individual innovators in a conference working session. These professionals generally find themselves, by choice, overcommitted and often unavailable for ''just one more meeting.'' This conference was designed to pull the participants out of their usual settings and place them on a practice-oriented turf. For the health delivery system, it seems crucial that every step be taken to encourage the interchange between those who are involved in research and development leading to change and those responsible for implementation of change.

The book explores this topic of merging financial and clinical systems; it will be evident that such a tour through a very complex subject is beneficial.

In the past, data processing, to many, suggested the mechanization of health care. To those involved in the present and the future, an understanding of how organized and integrated data usage can affect positively the delivery of higher quality and more effective health care is crucial.

Austin Ross

Chapter 1

Data for Case-Mix Management: Status and Future Prospects

Gerald E. Bisbee, Jr., and *Marilyn P. Plomann*

The growth in the volume and specificity of information required to manage the hospital and report to payers and regulators has paralleled the increase in hospital revenue. Information is data that have been evaluated for their worth; the data necessary to produce the increasing information demanded have grown in both quantity and quality. The 1983 amendments to the Social Security Act (P.L. 98-21) require that hospitals be paid based on their diagnosis related group (DRG) mix. This requirement virtually guarantees that hospitals will refine existing financial, administrative, and clinical data bases and merge them in order to understand and control the financial and clinical activities of the institution, thereby further increasing its data needs.

HOSPITAL DATA REQUIREMENTS

Before this century, hospital data were required so that the trustees knew how much to contribute to the institution at the end of the year. When the third party source of payment initiated by Blue Cross in the 1930s became more prevalent, new streams of fiscal, administrative, and patient-specific data were required to document the facility's activities. The Joint Commission on the Accreditation of Hospitals formalized the amount and type of clinical information an accredited hospital must collect. The Medicare and Medicaid regulations significantly increased the data collection requirements for both fiscal and clinical information, although no incentive was provided to integrate these data.

Sophisticated planning and budgeting in health care institutions traditionally was constrained by the lack of output to which revenues and expenses could be matched.[1] The absence of adequate output measures was the primary reason why management control was more difficult in health care institutions than in organizations with identifiable products.

Historically, accounting techniques for planning and control were developed in manufacturing rather than nonmanufacturing firms because the measurement problems were less imposing, i.e., there was a definable unit of output that served as the basis of the accounting system. Without this definable unit, the basis for responsibility accounting, variance analysis, and control of operating expenses could not exist. Planning and management control in institutions with definable products is complicated by the existence of more than one product; thus, health care institutions that clearly are multiproduct firms and do not have readily definable products have sophisticated information and data needs.

The solution to defining hospitals' output or product, which has been studied by researchers for years, has relied on the merger of clinical and financial data in order to equate the dollar flows with the purpose of the facilities' existence, i.e., to provide clinical services to patients. A complete analysis of related research is found elsewhere and is not reviewed extensively here.[2] To summarize the literature briefly, the merger of clinical and financial data for purposes of describing hospitals' output includes initial work by Martin Feldstein,[3] study in Europe on what was called "disease costing,"[4] and the work of Riedel and Fitzpatrick as part of the Hospital and Medical Economics study project conducted in the early 1960s at the University of Michigan.[5]

Riedel's early work led to the development of the DRG at Yale University by Thompson and Fetter. Since the original purpose of DRGs was utilization review, data collection focused on clinical and utilization variables. Major funding for DRG development from the Social Security Administration and later the Health Care Financing Administration was directed to the use of DRGs for payment of hospitals under Medicare.

In 1980-1983, the Hospital Research and Educational Trust, under a grant funded by the W. K. Kellogg Foundation and the Duke Endowment, created a planning, budgeting, and clinical management system based on integrated financial and clinical data streams of the hospital.

The 1983 prospective payment legislation changed the prevailing mode of Medicare payment from retrospective, cost-based reimbursement to prospective payment. This clearly is the greatest change in the financing of hospital care since Medicare and Medicaid became effective in 1966 and has the potential for fundamentally altering the relationship among physicians, hospitals, and patients. Hospital leaders were galvanized to act to increase the management control capabilities of their institutions. Underlying any case-mix management reporting system is a merged clinical and financial data base. The rest of this chapter addresses the issues relating to the present and future data needs required by case-mix management systems in hospitals.

USE OF DATA AND RELATED ISSUES

This section discusses the use of data for case-mix systems for purposes of management and finance, clinical applications, and both institutional and community planning.

Management and Finance

To compete most effectively in the increasingly demanding health care environment, hospital leaders are taking a longer term view of management and increasingly are including case-mix information based on integrated clinical and financial information in their resource allocation decision making.

Research by the Trust in the design, development, and demonstration of an integrated clinical and financial management system reveals six data-related factors that need to be addressed before the system will realize its full potential:

1. quality of clinical data
2. quantity of data for operational analysis
3. methods for determining cost
4. integration of data streams
5. comparability of information across hospitals
6. selection of appropriate definition of hospital product

Each of these factors is discussed next.

Quality of Clinical Data

Two important studies that address the issue of data quality and reliability were conducted by the Institute of Medicine (IOM) in 1975[6] and by the Health Research and Educational Trust of New Jersey (New Jersey) in 1977.[7] These studies found that nonmedical data items, e.g., admission and discharge dates, date of birth, sex, and payment source, were highly reliable. However, much less reliability was shown for diagnostic and procedural information:

- For principal diagnosis, the IOM reabstract corresponded to the original abstract in 65.2 percent of the records, while the New Jersey study found that the principal diagnosis was reliable in 72.6 percent.
- Both studies found that the more complex the diagnosis, the higher the discrepancy rate. For example, the IOM study reported no discrepancies in 94.3 percent of the records for patients with cataracts, 60.8 percent for diabetes mellitus, and 30.2 percent for chronic ischemic heart disease.
- In terms of procedures, the IOM study indicated that the overall level of agreement between abstracted and reabstracted data was 73.2 percent. In the New Jersey study, the level of reliability for principal procedures was 66.4 percent and for all other procedures 59.3 percent.

A medical record discharge abstracting study of all six demonstration hospitals in Washington was conducted as part of the Trust's Planning, Budgeting and Clinical Management Project (PBCS).[8] The study was designed to assess (1) the reliability of demographic and clinical information used in management reports and (2) the effect of assignment of patients to DRG categories.

1. Reliability of Demographic and Clinical Information. The PBCS study found a high accuracy rate among abstracted nonmedical data similar to the other studies. Errors that did occur were caused primarily by clerical errors. In the case of clinical data, the PBCS hospitals' overall accuracy rate in identifying the principal diagnosis was 79 percent, the accuracy rate for principal procedures 84 percent.

These studies were conducted at different times with different methodologies and data bases. However, as shown in Table 1–1, the results from all three are relatively similar, with the PBCS study finding higher accuracy rates than the two others for two reasons:

1. The International Classification of Diseases-9 (ICD-9) codes were used for the PBCS study, ICD-8 codes for the IOM and New Jersey studies. The ICD-9 is a newer, more refined coding system and a higher accuracy rate would be expected.
2. The demonstration hospitals had a stronger incentive for accuracy, given their involvement in the study.

For diagnostic and procedural information, errors stemmed most frequently from difficulty in determining which diagnosis should be regarded as principal. Many hospitals routinely select the first diagnosis listed on the face sheet of the medical record as the principal diagnosis, regardless of additional documentation. The major reason for discrepancies (both coding and diagnosis sequencing) was failure to review the medical record adequately before designating a principal diagnosis and/or principal procedure. Other reasons included:

- The medical record was incomplete at the time it was coded, causing an admitting or provisional diagnosis to be used.
- The face sheet, discharge summary, and/or operative report may have been unavailable.

Table 1–1 Accuracy Rate by Study

Study	Principal Diagnosis	Principal Procedure
IOM	65.2	73.2
New Jersey	72.6	66.4
PBCS	78.9	83.7

• Diagnoses may have been added, deleted, modified, or resequenced after coders completed the abstract.

2. Effect of Assignment of Patients to DRGs. In terms of the assignment of patients to the correct DRG, Table 1-2 indicates the percentage of reabstracted records that changed major diagnostic categories (MDCs) and DRG assignments because of discrepancies in one or more of the DRG-related data items. About one out of five records was assigned to the incorrect DRG in the PBCS study because of coding errors and discrepancies in selection of the principal diagnosis. As would be expected, the more general MDC category had a lower percentage of incorrect assignments.

This incorrect assignment is not related to ''DRG drift'' that has been discussed as a strategy hospitals might pursue to increase their revenue. Rather this incorrect assignment is caused by errors. Since DRGs give hospitals a financial incentive to ensure that data are error free, the discrepancy rate will decline.[9,10] The rules and regulations under the prospective payment legislation[11] also address an important cause of error—sequencing of the identification of illness. The regulations require that the attending physician attest to the principal diagnosis and procedures in writing before a claim is submitted. This probably will increase the accuracy rate.

Quantity of Data for Operational Analysis

As financial pressures on hospitals increase, more data—both management and clinical—will be collected and analyzed. For example, answers will be sought to the following questions:

• How are physician practice patterns related to training, background, and specialty?
• What are the health statuses of patients upon admission?
• What is the relative efficiency of a hospital's use of resources to produce a specific service?

Table 1-2 Incorrect Assignment Because of Data Discrepancies

Assignment Category	Percentage of Total Records
MDC	8.2
DRG	20.2

- What are specific regional differences in case type?
- What are differences in severity among patients with the same diagnosis?

The specificity of billing and clinical information varies from hospital to hospital. Highly nonspecific data limit managers' ability to pinpoint differences in practice patterns and their financial impact. Without detailed data, clinicians or managers cannot assess causes of financial or quality variances.

One area requiring more specific data is the room-and-board category of hospital expense. This consists of a number of expenses that are difficult to allocate directly to individual patients. Nursing is the largest room-and-board element. In 1982, nursing was 18.2 percent of total cost per day and 36.5 percent of salary cost per day. The capability of analyzing nursing productivity and relating it to particular DRGs is a major challenge for future research and development activities.[12]

In summary, hospitals with highly specific billing and clinical information have a head start on operational analysis that is a necessity for management of hospitals in today's rapidly changing environment.

Methods for Determining Cost

Financial information includes both charge and cost data. The billing system records the charges for services and the cost-accounting system the expense of providing care. The most accurate source of such information is a cost-accounting system that is detailed enough to collect specific data. Two methods of approximating cost can be used with a case-mix system: (1) ratio of cost to charges and (2) procedural costing. A discussion of each follows.

1. Ratio of Cost to Charges (RCC). The RCC is available from the Medicare cost report and can be used for Medicare and non-Medicare patients. However, more refined information is available if a unique cost-to-charge ratio is calculated for each payer. The RCC is easily available and requires no additional cost or effort to produce. The Medicare cost report is required by law through 1988, although it probably will continue in some form as long as services such as outpatient care and pass-throughs (i.e., capital, research, and medical education) are not covered by a prospective rate.

The RCC is not as accurate as procedural costing because:

- Departmental ratios are dependent upon the step-down allocation method regulated by Medicare.
- Ratios are based on historical relationships that may not reflect current cost.
- Ratios are available at the cost center level only; costs of individual procedures and tests cannot be identified.
- Ratios reflect cross-subsidization of different units.

Even with these drawbacks, the RCC is a necessary beginning to assessing cost in the absence of a sophisticated cost-accounting system.

2. Procedural Costing. This method uses a more refined, precise approach to determine the costs of a particular procedure or service. While it does provide the most accurate cost information for each element, it requires a commitment from the hospital in terms of time and resources.

The overall approach to developing procedure cost is to allocate the actual (or budgeted) direct and indirect costs of each revenue-producing cost center to each of the services it produces. To accomplish this, it is necessary first to segregate costs into a number of components, such as direct labor, indirect labor, capital, etc. These components then are allocated to the individual procedures, using an appropriate set of relative value units (RVUs) for each component. RVUs attempt to measure the relative amount of resources consumed by each procedure, as compared with all other procedures. RVUs can be hospital specific by defining them through interviews with departmental heads or time studies, or they can represent national values such as the laboratory CAP (College of American Pathologists) values.

Procedure costs need to be identified as fixed or variable. This will enable the hospital to simulate the impact of different volume levels and pricing strategies on profitability by patient, program, and payer. Fixed costs do not vary with the level of output, whereas variable costs do fluctuate as tests, procedures, or daily stays increase or decrease. The individual fixed and variable components that comprise the total cost, and thus need to be identified and calculated for each procedure, are:

1. professional labor—fixed
2. administrative labor—fixed
3. direct labor—variable (technicians, nurses, etc.)
4. supplies—variable
5. equipment—fixed
6. service overhead—fixed (e.g., travel, relocation, etc.)
7. support centers—fixed or variable (e.g., housekeeping, engineering, etc.)

Development of costs by these components allows management to enhance the quality of its decision making.

Integration of Data Streams

Historically, integrating clinical and financial data has been expensive and time consuming because of the large volumes of data required. The increased capabilities of computers have eliminated their capacity as a problem. Large hospitals can afford computers with enough capacity to merge their data bases.

Similarly, the large data processing services also can integrate data for hospitals that do not have their own computer capability.

The software required for integrating clinical and financial data can be expensive to write. Technical difficulties can arise regarding unique patient identifiers for each data stream. These problems generally are solvable, particularly if the data are accurate.

Comparability of Information Across Hospitals

An important management tool is provided the hospital when it is able to compare its revenues and expenses with those of other similar facilities. In terms of case-mix data, comparability is complicated by the normal differences in hospital organization and data quality and quantity and in standard definitions for particular cases. The DRG is an important initial step in comparing hospitals' performance. The complexity of individual cases within a DRG may vary across hospitals, which will confound the comparison. For example, if Hospital A uses more resources for a given DRG than does Hospital B, the differences may involve efficiency, practice patterns, severity of illness, etc.

For reason of necessity, dollars have been used as a substitute for services utilized. Charges or costs are not as specific a measure of the use of routine and ancillary department services as is the number and type of tests or services.

Selection of Appropriate Definition of Hospital Product

Researchers have approached the definition of the hospital's product by using a measure of the case mix as a proxy. For example, each DRG could be considered a product. The prospective payment legislation causes hospital managers to adopt a product orientation to planning and budgeting their resources.

Each case-mix classification system will define the product mix of the hospital somewhat differently because each system was designed for a different purpose and utilizes a different methodology. There are nine classification systems, which are described in detail elsewhere.[13]

The particular data elements used by each of the case-mix classification systems vary significantly. For example, the systems intended for quality assurance applications focus on measuring the severity of disease, and each uses many different data elements or patient characteristics to evaluate that factor. Each system possesses strengths and weaknesses that should be considered before being applied in the hospital setting. The purpose of development of the system should be related to the objectives for its use.

Case-mix groups are a common basis for administrators and physicians to plan and allocate resources. Therefore, the case-mix categories must be meaningful to both groups and reflect the resources available in the hospital.

Most existing classification systems require some degree of modification to create case-mix groups that are useful to a given hospital's administrative and medical staffs. The systems may need to be refined for several reasons:

- Each was developed originally for a specific purpose.
- Each used a different patient population that may not totally reflect the client types found in a particular institution.
- Each was designed to explain other variables such as length of stay or total charges rather than the spectrum of resources allocated by hospital managers and physicians.

Clinical Applications

The use of case-mix information systems for clinical applications is addressed in Chapter 4, by Joseph Gonnella and Carter Zeleznik, so this discussion focuses mainly on data limitations and how they relate to clinical applications.

In the past, clinical practices were analyzed to meet utilization review and quality assurance requirements. Subsequent legislation reinforced these activities. The Tax Equity and Fiscal Responsibility Act of 1982 (TEFRA) (P.L. 97-248) created the Peer Review Improvement Act of 1982. The legislation repealed the professional standards review organization (PSRO) program and created in its place a program in which the Department of Health and Human Services enters into agreements with peer review organizations (PROs) to form utilization and quality control peer review.

The PROs focus on:

- the validity of diagnostic information provided by the hospital
- the completeness, accuracy, and quality of care provided
- the appropriateness of admissions and discharges
- the appropriateness of care for which additional payments are sought beyond the DRG prospective payment rate.

Given the increasing fiscal incentives to monitor practice patterns, the utilization and quality assurance program then becomes part of the overall management strategy to control costs. The hospital allocates more resources to increasing the quality and quantity of its data.

The most effective utilization review program is one that is conducted concurrently and is focused on unique utilization patterns by DRG, physician, and payer. A clinical/financial information system can assist in this process by:

- providing information on past utilization patterns for developing acceptable protocols and ranges of resource use
- identifying cases that fall outside the standard.

However, since most integrated systems are based on the medical record abstracts, they cannot support concurrent review. Other limiting factors include:

- The quality of clinical data: If the data are not valid, physicians will have no confidence in them and will find them of limited use for a focused review program.
- The quantity of clinical and financial data on the medical record abstract: This can limit physicians' ability to define clinical protocols for disease categories.

The discharge abstract data set does not provide sufficient information to define disease categories that are medically meaningful for development of protocols. A medical diagnosis should include information documenting the manifestations, severity, location, and cause of the patient's problem.[14] Although used as a basis for payment, DRGs never were intended to represent treatment protocols, hence their clinical applicability is limited. DRGs do not reflect disease etiology, the organ system affected, or the severity of the patient's condition.

Two studies discussed next compared the medical record with the discharge abstract in relation to assigning cases to case-mix categories. The results show that the abstract is less useful than the chart for accurately and completely defining case-mix categories, primarily because the abstract has less complete information than the chart.

One of the two studies, by the National Center for Health Services Research,[15] assessed the difference between assigning a patient to a disease stage using the complete medical record or using automated discharge abstract data with staging software. Using abstract data, there was an overall match rate (patient assigned to same stage under both conditions) of 77.4 percent. The match rate varied by coding system:

- International Classification of Diseases A-8 (72.1 percent)
- Hospital Adaptation of International Classification of Diseases A-2 (76.9 percent)
- International Classification of Diseases-9-Clinical Modification (80.6 percent).

The International Classification of Diseases-9-Clinical Modification system generally produced better results because of the increased specificity in the diagnostic coding. The match rates also varied across disease groups, with high rates for newborns and birth trauma/disease (99.9 percent) and low rates for hemiparesis and reticuloendothelial (38.9 percent).

In all these diseases, the reasons for discrepancies between manual and machine staging were as shown in Table 1–3.

In the second study, conducted by the Health Care Research Department of Blue Cross of Western Pennsylvania,[16] similar results were found. This study used a different classification system, Patient Management Categories, but assessed the difference between a computerized method of patient assignment using data available on discharge abstracts versus manual assignments based on complete medical records. In 4,348 cases, there was a match rate of 72 percent between the two methods. When the discharge abstracts were corrected for errors in assignment of principal diagnosis, coding of diagnosis, omission and exclusion of codes, the match rate was 90 percent.

Managers, in addition to having limited clinical data for defining disease groups, may find the financial data do not provide the level of detail necessary to provide a profile of past resource use for identifying acceptable clinical protocols. Hospitals will find it cost effective to enhance current billing systems to capture the data needed for detailed analysis.

An integrated system also can assist in the monitoring of quality care by the incorporation of additional existing clinical data streams in hospitals, such as nosocomial infection reports, pathology reports, and incidence reports.

Planning

Hospital decision makers no longer operate in an environment of unlimited financial resources and public enthusiasm for expansion and modernization. The current environment requires significantly increased planning mechanisms that consider hospitals' goals and employ mechanisms for evaluating their performance.[17]

Table 1–3 Reasons for Discrepancies Between Manual and Machine
      Staging

Understated:	
Lack of ICD-9-CM Code Specificity	33.6%
Complications not coded (includes laboratory values not collected) on original discharge abstract	52.6%
Death status conflict	0%
Overstated:	
Complications coded that were not found in chart on reabstract	12.1%
Death status conflict	0%
Misinterpretation of staging terminology	1.7%

Institutional planning within hospitals has grown in sophistication in recent years, as each facility has had to compete with other institutions and forms of delivery. More sophisticated planning activities include segmenting the hospital's market by age, location, and type of services used. With the advent of DRGs and other case-mix measures, institutional planning has segmented its community by case-mix category. The main data requirements are case-mix information on the community and extension of case types to the entire community population using epidemiological concepts.

Operational and capital planning can become more sophisticated by use of product-oriented analysis based on case-mix measures, as suggested earlier in this chapter. Many of the capabilities of planning, budgeting, and control systems that are found in industry are applicable to hospitals if DRGs or other case-mix measures are used as products.

Community-based planning has not been particularly effective in the United States. Availability of DRG information may provide community planning agencies with another dimension of information for influencing the allocation of hospital resources. The standard incidence, prevalence, and patient origin information must be updated for particular DRGs. This requires substantial resources and study by epidemiologists and health service researchers.

FUTURE DIRECTIONS

The advent of prospective pricing under Medicare for inpatient hospital services has heightened the need for an integrated clinical and financial information system like PBCS. The new payment system creates an incentive to control costs for two reasons:

1. Prospective pricing places the institution at risk by not covering all of the expenses if the actual cost of providing health care exceeds the prescribed rate.
2. Prospective pricing allows the institution to retain part of the difference if the cost of care is lower than the prescribed payment for a given diagnosis.

These incentives require that hospital costs be examined according to how they are generated and, consequently, how they can be controlled on a per case basis.

With clear incentives now present for the measurement, monitoring, and improvement of hospital productivity, as well as for the development of productivity management programs, institutions need to address several key issues if they are to be economically successful under prospective pricing:

- Productivity Measurement: Before the prospective payment system (PPS), hospital productivity measurement systems were departmentally based. Progressive hospitals must investigate methods to provide productivity information using more than the DRG system mandated by the prospective pricing legislation. Increased attention must be paid to identifying and measuring the aggregation of services required to produce the hospital's case mix.

- Productivity Improvement: The "science" of improving productivity in hospitals must integrate the contributions of behavioral scientists and management engineers. New measurement techniques and work methods must be combined with concern for two-way communication between employees and management, and for worker motivation and work environment. An effective hospital productivity effort should involve all levels of labor and management as well as the medical staff and trustees.

- Quality Maintenance: Some skepticism exists as to the viability of transferring industrial concepts of productivity to hospitals. Medical and nursing staffs' concerns for the quality of patient care must be addressed as crucial elements of any hospital productivity program. Quality assurance mechanisms need to be monitored and strengthened in the face of incentives to reduce overall hospital costs.

- Hospital Organization: The role of physicians and nurses in hospital management decisions regarding productivity is not well defined. Innovative models and methods for administration, medical staff, and nursing service collaboration on productivity issues need to be identified and evaluated.

In sum, hospitals have made substantial progress throughout this century in their use of data for management and clinical purposes. This has been particularly true since the 1950s. DRGs and other case-mix measures present a new opportunity for hospitals to further refine their planning, budgeting, and clinical management systems.

The prospective payment system clearly increases hospitals' incentive to integrate financial and clinical data, which thereby increases the quality and quantity of both types of data. Error rates should decrease as hospitals and physicians have the financial incentive to improve the quality of the institution's data.

More study is needed on determining the true costs of hospital care by DRG. This involves the breakdown of routine costs so that they may be allocated to specific patients and DRGs. More study also is needed on the use of clinical data in management decisions and how best to refine the data collection systems.

NOTES

1. G.E. Bisbee, "The Relationship Between Case Mix and the Management and Allocation of Medical Care Resources" (Ph.D. diss., Yale University, 1974).

2. Ibid.

3. Martin S. Feldstein, "Hospital Cost Variation and Case-Mix Differences," *Medical Care* 3:95.

4. J.H. Babson, *Disease Costing* (Manchester, England: Manchester University Press, 1973).

5. W.J. McNerney et al., *Hospital and Medical Economics* (Chicago: Hospital Research and Educational Trust, 1962).

6. L.K. Demlo, P.M. Campbell et al., "Reliability of Information Abstracted from Patients' Medical Records," *Medical Care* (December 1978).

7. Health Research and Educational Trust of New Jersey, *Reliability of New Jersey Hospital Discharge Abstracts* (Trenton: New Jersey Department of Health, 1978).

8. "Reliability of 1981 Hospital Discharge Abstracts from Planning, Budgeting, and Control Project Participating Hospitals" (Chicago: Hospital Research and Educational Trust, 1982).

9. Bisbee, "Relationship."

10. "Reliability."

11. *Federal Register* 48, no. 171.

12. Office of Public Policy Analysis and Hospital Administrative Services, American Hospital Association, 1982.

13. M.P. Plomann, *Case-Mix Classification Systems: Development, Description, and Testing* (Chicago: Hospital Research and Educational Trust, 1982).

14. J.S. Gonnella, "Patient Case Mix: Implications for Medical Education and Hospital Costs," *Journal of Medical Education* 56 (1981): 610–11.

15. National Center for Health Services Research, Hospital Cost and Utilization Project, Contract No. 233-78-3001.

16. W.W. Young et al., "The Measurement of Hospital Case Mix," *Medical Care*.

17. *Environmental Assessment Overview: 1983* (Chicago: Hospital Research and Educational Trust, 1983).

Chapter 2

Financial Issues in the Integration of Clinical and Financial Data Systems

Truman H. Esmond, Jr.

In 1976, this writer became the chief financial officer of a major medical center and for the next six years worked with some marvelous people analyzing the condition of the health care industry, modeling and planning for the future. Much of what it was possible to determine indicated that the industry's fortunes were going to deteriorate. Although this group predicted gloom and doom, the patient days and the profitability of the institution and many others remained right on target, year after year. As a result, at least in this institution, it appeared that some in the group were losing credibility.

A look back on those years indicates that the analysis and predictions were right. The fortunes of the industry were not as good as had been thought and they have gotten worse. During that boom period in the late 1970s, the industry was borrowing to finance more and more of the same at ever higher prices. Many referred to it then as growth. Table 2–1 indicates how much growth there really was.[1]

These statistics indicate that the growth was not in admissions or in inpatient days; it was primarily in operating expenses. Most new construction was financed with debt. In 1968, debt accounted for 38.2 percent of a community hospital's construction expenditures. By 1981, that figure had risen to 75.8 percent.[2] The average funding per construction project in that period jumped 153.8 percent. The constant dollar value of the average funding per project during the same period actually increased by 33.8 percent,[3] which indicates that a substantial portion of total borrowing was required just to cover inflation.

Normally, this increase in capital costs over historic depreciation would be covered by growth in net income. Figures 2–1 and 2–2 indicate the condition of net income during that period.[4,5] Instead of generating capital from current income, hospital managers were borrowing more to cover inflated capital costs, putting increased pressure on future income.

During this period, hospitals were paying relatively high interest rates considering that they were able to borrow on the tax-exempt market. Underwriters and

Table 2–1 Selected Community Hospital Statistics

	1977	1978	1979	1980	1981	1982	1983	% Change (Decrease) 1977-1983
Utilization Data:								
Hospitals	5,881	5,851	5,842	5,830	5,813	5,801	5,783	(1.7%)
Admissions (millions)	34.2	34.5	35.1	36.1	36.4	36.4	36.2	5.8%
Inpatient Days (millions)	261.0	262.1	265.4	272.7	278.5	278.1	273.4	4.8%
Adult Length of Stay (days)	7.6	7.6	7.6	7.6	7.6	7.6	7.6	0%
Outpatient Visits (millions)	198.7	201.9	198.8	202.3	202.8	248.1	210.0	5.7%
Beds (thousands)	969	975	984	988	1,003	1,012	1,018	5.1%
Adult Occupancy Rate	73.8%	73.6%	73.9%	75.6%	76.0%	75.3%	73.5%	.4%
Operating Expense Data:								
Total (billions)	$51.6	$58.2	$66.0	$76.9	$90.6	$104.9	$116.4	125.6%
Inpatient Expense per Admission	$1,322	$1,474	$1,642	$1,851	$2,171	$2,500	$2,789	111.0%
Total Hospital Payroll (billions)	$25.9	$28.9	$32.6	$37.4	$44.0	$50.6	$55.5	114.3%

Source: *Hospital Statistics*, p. 7, American Hospital Association, © 1984.

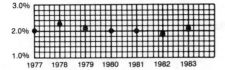

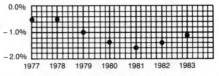

Figure 2–1 Hospital Net Income as a Percentage of Total Operating Revenue

Source: The Hospital Industry Analysis Report 1981, Healthcare Financial Management Association, © 1983.

Figure 2–2 Hospital Net Income as a Percentage of Total Operating Revenue *(Price Level Adjusted)*

Source: The Hospital Industry Analysis Report 1981, Healthcare Financial Management Association, © 1983.

---

bankers were encouraging debt, pointing out that, compared with utility companies and airlines, hospitals had tremendous unused debt capacity. In 1981, for example, community hospitals had a debt-to-assets ratio of 44 percent, as compared to 61 percent for utilities and 73 percent for airlines.

By 1983 many analysts were saying that the hospital industry had reached its capacity to borrow. They now point to the low profit margin, the relatively poor outlook for government payment programs, the few government grants for capital, and the decrease in philanthropy. The bankers, the underwriters, and hospital financial managers were coming to the same conclusion: the industry's financial condition was eroding.

The purpose here is to analyze the condition as of 1983, project where future government payment will take the industry, and identify the specific changes that must take place in administrative departments within individual organizations.

BACKGROUND OF THE SITUATION

Compared with the "good old days" of the 1970s, times were not good in 1983, and were to get worse. The managers of the hospital industry found themselves in an environment of increasing costs, greater public awareness, tighter government regulations, and decreasing financial viability. At the same time, many managers were making it worse by continuing practices that had led to their dilemma. They were attempting to provide all services to all people. They were borrowing to provide capital—some even borrowing to provide working capital. Their institutions were generating an inadequate bottom line (they were truly "nonprofit"). They were offsetting government underpayment by overcharging other patients. They were looking to nonoperating revenue for survival and hoping that the recent hospital reorganization and the formation of a for-profit subsidiary would provide the necessary revenue to build a strong institution.

Significant changes obviously were in the making. Management had to adapt if their institutions were to get by, and even prosper, with fewer resources. Not many institutions were expected to go out of business but many nursing units were likely to be closed and the role of many institutions would change. For some, even the nature of the business would change. The way to success in the 1983 environment involved looking at institutions as businesses as well as social entities. The two concepts are not incompatible. Communities have entrusted hospitals with assets in some cases of more than $10 million, in other cases of more than $100 million. The institutions thus had a responsibility to utilize those assets properly, which meant following sound business practices. In an era of reduced resources, managers had to prioritize the resource requirements.

Administrators had to identify their product (program output) in relation to their mission. It was necessary to eliminate some programs or product lines that were not compatible with that mission or that simply could not be afforded any longer. By eliminating programs that were draining their resources, hospitals could focus their remaining resources and even expand or improve the quality of other programs. Quality became the new guideline. Payers knew they could obtain services at low prices but could not determine value (the quality/price trade-off) because they had not been able to define quality. Once they could focus on the treated patient as the primary product, they could turn their attention to the definition, measurement, and management of quality. Hospitals then had to tell the public about their institutions and the services they offered, using sophisticated communication marketing techniques. Lastly, they had to concentrate on the bottom line, the net income, for long-term financial viability.

THE SITUATION IN THE MID-1980s

The situation in 1983 was confusing. It was clear that major third party payers had reduced the resources they would make available. Several years earlier, the state of Illinois Medicaid program was a skimpy, grossly underfunded system. The governor in effect said, "Go ahead, hospital managers, provide the services to the Medicaid recipients and trust me for the balance due." The hospitals reacted by instituting a lawsuit to ensure that the plan would be funded. The hospitals won. The state requested bids from hospitals for contracts for payment on a capitation basis to reduce expenditures. Few contracts were signed. The state then asked for bids on a per diem basis. Most hospitals in Illinois that serve Medicaid patients contracted for fewer days at a reduced per diem.

Medicare cut back on hospital payments nationally and introduced the concept of budget neutrality to ensure savings of $813 million in 1983, $1.866 billion in

1984, and \$3.5 billion in 1985. A study by the Congressional Budget Office, however, showed that this was not enough.[6] As Table 2–2 indicates, the hospital insurance trust fund faced a deficit position by 1987 that was expected to increase to \$401 billion by 1995.

The timing of the crossover into a deficit position was widely discussed and restudied. (Don Moran, executive associate director, Office of Management and Budget, in 1985 indicated the positive balance could last as long as late 1989, depending upon sustained growth of the economy.[7]) As pointed out by Ginsburg and Curtis, the options available to Medicare to correct the situation were drastic:[8]

1. to substantially increase the coinsurance for all Medicare patients
2. to hold hospital price boosts to a negative real increase
3. to expand the fund balance by substantially increasing the hospital insurance payroll tax
4. to fund the deficits from general revenues
5. to combine some or all of these.

In the author's view, any attempt to keep the trust fund out of a deficit position eventually would include copayment for Medicare patients, which would mean

Table 2–2 Projections of Hospital Insurance Trust Fund Outlays, Income, and Balances

(By Calendar Year—In Billions of Dollars)

Year	Outlays	Income	Year-End Balance
1981	\$30.7	\$35.7	\$18.7
1982	36.0	25.6	8.3
1983	41.1	41.6	8.8
1984	46.2	44.8	7.4
1985	51.0	49.5	5.9
1986	60.0	56.3	2.2
1987	68.5	59.7	−6.5
1988	77.0	63.1	−20.4
1989	86.6	66.3	−40.7
1990	97.4	69.2	−68.9
1991	109.5	71.7	−106.7
1992	123.0	73.5	−156.3
1993	138.2	74.7	−219.8
1994	155.4	75.1	−300.1
1995	174.8	74.1	−400.9

Source: Adapted from *Health Affairs*, pp. 102–111, with permission of Project HOPE, © Spring 1983.

reduced hospital utilization—shorter stays and fewer admissions. It is time for a new type of compromise, one that, for the first time, includes taking something away from Medicare beneficiaries. Benefits and/or flexibility must be limited, which in turn would decrease demand for facilities even further.

Other payers attempted to lower health care costs by negotiating discounts, reducing employee benefits, and introducing legislation at the state level to control hospital pricing. Blue Cross, a major payer in this group, in several states mandated capitation—predetermined payments based upon diagnosis related groups (DRGs) or negotiated rates.

A concomitant was the rapid growth of a whole new group known as the Medicare poor. As deductibles and copayment increased, this group was differentiated from the Medicare insured or Medicare self-pay group. These patients would become increasingly important to the inner city hospitals and those with high Medicare utilization.

What major payers did in the past is important, but what they will do in the future is far more important. It is clear that payer financing problems will result in reduced utilization. In Chicago, the impact of reduced utilization was felt early. By 1979, utilization had begun to fall and by 1983 had not turned around despite major efforts. In the next half-dozen years, utilization was expected to get worse, largely because of changes by Medicare and other major third party payers. As a result of these reduced resources, there was tremendous competition among hospitals and alternative delivery systems for patients, particularly for those who were willing and able to pay for services.

The confusing factor in all this gloom and doom is that many institutions had been experiencing relatively profitable years. The trustees and medical staffs found it hard to believe that times were tough when profits were relatively good. What they were seeing, however, did not prove that times were not tough; it just proved that they still could maintain a bottom line by raising prices and being a little cost conscious. Hospitals knew, however, that this strategy would not continue to work in the future because their ability to raise prices was limited.

THE FUTURE: WHAT IS THE ANSWER?

After discussing the past and analyzing the present, the real focus must be on the future. Hospitals cannot change what happens today and, for the most part, what will happen next month. Primarily because of the nature of their services and the time it takes to implement change, hospitals need to focus on the next year or the next three years.

Trends in 1983 indicated more competition from alternative delivery systems, empty beds, and an acceptance of more risk by health providers. The number of health maintenance organizations (HMOs) grew 15.3 percent in 1983, after a few years of slowing growth. The number of persons enrolled in HMOs was predicted to continue to increase as more employers looked for an alternative to pay-as-you-use-it hospital coverage. (The average length of stay dropped from 7.2 days in the first quarter of 1983 to 6.7 days in the first quarter of 1985. Total admissions fell 8.7 percent in the same period. The hospital inpatient days per thousand population were declining and the industry was not sure where utilization would stabilize.)

The market for the sale and purchase of hospital services was projected to change significantly over time. In 1985, managers sold hospital services to a "wholesale" market—major third parties, which packaged the services and resold them to employers. The packages took a number of forms to suit employer needs. Many companies offer employees one or more alternative delivery systems as options to traditional insurance coverage. As more options are made available, it will benefit hospitals or groups of them to join with other providers and sell directly to employees. This eliminates the middle man and providers, if necessary, can carry the risk related to the amount and type of usage of health care facilities. This direct selling, or "retail," type of market will be facilitated by consumers' increased knowledge concerning the delivery of care and the use of vouchers to provide them with the flexibility to choose from a broad range of providers and types of coverage. This retail market might function as follows:

- The employer would set certain criteria that providers must meet in order to be "qualified."
- The employer then would give each employee a voucher that would obligate the employer for a preestablished amount of dollars per month.
- The employees, armed with these vouchers, would be free to choose from among the various options, to supplement the vouchers with their own funds, to purchase a luxury package, or to use the savings obtained from the purchase of a limited hospital plan (a larger deductible, for example) to acquire other benefits.

This type of market will be encouraged more by the health care providers than by employers as the former seek to obtain insurance profits and move to serve a greater portion of their community. Of course, once the retail market is working for employers, the government will provide vouchers for Medicare and Medicaid recipients and allow them to select from a long list of qualified providers. As the industry moves away from the traditional third party payer role, it will be developing a totally new set of relationships, responsibilities, and risks.

Among the providers there will be those who accept the risk related to demand and pricing and those who subcontract to risk takers to provide care on the traditional per-visit, per-day, or per-case basis. The successful risk takers will prosper and all subcontractor providers will continue to feel the squeeze.

Where can the answers be found? Where can administrators locate a successful model? Can they copy what other industries have done? They have tried this in the past:

- They have looked at manufacturing companies and found that it is easier to manufacture radiology equipment than to utilize it effectively.
- They have looked at hotels, but patients are not in hospitals on a vacation or in town on business.
- They have looked at the food service industry but have found that it is harder to prepare and deliver three warm, nutritious meals to patients' rooms than to operate a fast-food carryout.

Administrators' jobs are difficult, but they have made their tasks more difficult because they have not been able to focus resources as well as their counterparts in other industries. They need to target resources where they count, to increase their skill at focusing, and to improve their ability to predict expected results. They must concentrate on output and outcome.

Therefore, rather than looking at what their counterparts do in other industries, hospital leaders must ascertain how they do it. In looking again at those other industries, what do health care executives see? They see the power of profit—the difference it makes in the abilities of managers to utilize resources successfully because they can focus on priority goals. Even without a comprehensive strategic plan, managers can analyze challenges in terms of profit potential. A whole set of management and measurement tools has been developed around profit, such as return on investment, payback, ratio analysis, etc. Management can be given incentives to perform successfully with benefits such as stock options and profit sharing. Hospitals must have goals to guide their activities. Those goals must be as clear to health care administrators as profit is to their counterparts in other industries.

In the past, hospitals did not develop those goals themselves. To a large extent, they were guided by third party payers. The government stressed access, and its payment policy followed political promises. The hospital industry responded successfully and provided new and better facilities to help ensure that access. Based on the adequacy of the payment, institutions made decisions to stay in relatively underserved areas and to provide a full range of services to the large portions of the population covered by government programs.

The government then suddenly shifted to divergent goals of access and low costs. The payment policy no longer is following the original political promises. Promises of access are being made, but hospitals no longer are being paid to provide those services. Hospital managers were not sure how to respond. In the era of PPS and DRGs, it is time for them to make decisions on their own, establishing goals to implement those decisions. Their difficult decisions concern access, price, and quality, because resources have been reduced and will be cut even more in the future.

What is the impact of reduced resources? How do executives operate in the short term? In the long term?

In the short term, they obviously must reduce costs and increase productivity. They could specialize or otherwise change the institution's role in the community. They could even alter the very nature of the institution from a hospital provider to an insurance company through contractual arrangements such as HMOs and capitation payments.

Every one of those possibilities offers potential or provides opportunity. Many managers are worried about mergers, takeovers, or the possiblity of having to sell out to an investor-owned system. The fact that any other organization is interested in that executive's institution means that someone believes that there still is potential in that community. A buyer looks for potential, for a turnaround situation. The "(HCA) figures that it takes up to five years to turn around a distressed institution and 18 months to raise a relatively healthy acquisition to a target level of profitability, which is an 18 percent pretax return on assets. . . ."[9]

Many sellers or hospitals looking for contract managers are doing so because they believe it will increase their access to capital. What is capital? It is no more than past or future profitability. If a large company is willing to provide an institution with access to the capital market, it means that the larger company sees potential in that hospital. Many institutions have the potential for a successful and financially sound future, but in order to take advantage of the opportunity managers must identify that potential and make the most of it.

The management of any given institution that has identified its potential and is making the most of it will have analyzed its strengths and weaknesses, identified its principal issues and problems, and established priorities. Such a management will have decided upon the institution's role in the delivery system and established a clear and understandable set of goals. It also will have included all this in an operating plan that clearly identifies the steps necessary to attain those goals, defines responsibilities, establishes a time frame for accomplishment of the goals, and gives the managers the tools to measure results. These seem like pretty lofty goals. Even if managers have accomplished all of these steps, there still may be some doubt as to the positive aspects of operating with reduced resources.

In the short term, steps must be taken in cost reduction. Administrators know that across-the-board cuts will not provide long-range results but that a reduction along program lines will. Analysis along product or program lines will help pick the correct spot for cutting. Reductions in some programs may provide the resources to strengthen others, thereby strengthening the institution as a whole.

As for productivity, having a time-study engineer follow a nurse or laboratory technician around the institution is not the answer. It is necessary to analyze the types of resources, personnel, and nonstaff personnel appropriate to support particular programs. Obviously, this type of analysis will focus attention on, for example, nursing—the number of nurses and the skills required. Nursing represents 16 to 19 percent of an institution's total cost, so the attention is warranted. This may lead management to develop more tailored basic care plans that rely on accommodation beds or home health programs to replace acute hospital utilization.

These efforts will lead to focusing resources on selected programs. As part of the overall analysis, management may well determine that the community will be better served if its institution focuses on some specific programs and its competitors on others.

THE CLINICAL/FINANCIAL DATA BASE

What tools do administrators need (in addition to imagination, leadership ability, and the full cooperation of the medical staff) to accomplish these changes? They must have good information, a good clinical/financial data base, program analysis capability that allows them to look at the hospital output in a variety of ways, and a strong operational plan to identify what is to be done, by whom, and when.

They also need a sound budget to allocate the resources in accordance with the operational plan. It is in the budget process that some of the first major changes will occur. As a result of the new management orientation, the budget must be program based. It should cover two years instead of only one. Managers know from experience that significant changes cannot be implemented in current programs, nor can they be added or deleted in a 12-month period. It is a great deal easier to discuss program alterations when analyzing the result of changes taking place two years hence. Because of this focus on programs, the budget process should change to target the second year instead of the first.

Specifically, the budget committee must determine what can be done over a two-year period, how it can be done, who will be responsible, and what resources will be required. Having determined what can be achieved by the end of the second year, the first-year budget becomes much easier to develop. Certain things must be done in the first year if the goals of the second year are to be accomplished, so specific directions are given for the first year. Specific responsibilities should be assigned so the individuals involved will have an easier time understanding the nature of their tasks.

At the end of the first year, the budget for the second year would be reviewed to make sure the assumptions were correct. The process then would focus on the second year, establishing new goals, making new assumptions, assigning updated responsibilities, and allocating resources.

The new budget must be flexible. In years past, managers could predict fairly accurately the statistics that provided the basis for a budget—the number of patient days and number of admissions. Since this no longer is true, they must control resources at various levels of activity. The new budget should provide for net income sufficient to cover capital requirements, working capital needs, and contingencies.

There also will be significant changes in the composition of the budget committee. Budgets used to be prepared by finance and administration working together. In many instances, physicians were asked for their input on a limited basis and, in some cases, were not asked at all. Future budgets will be prepared together with physicians who have the responsibilities for a specific program's success. That means physicians must accept responsibility in both the operating plan and in the budget if either is to be successful. As a result, physicians will come to make up a significant portion of the budget committee membership and participate in a new and better way to manage (and budget) resources. In some institutions, physicians are developing practice profiles that identify the services expected for specific patient groups. These profiles, together with current procedure level costing efforts, provide a sound basis for managing (and budgeting) resource requirements. This knowledge is another reason for physicians to participate actively and responsibly in the budget process.

WHERE DO ADMINISTRATORS BEGIN?

Where do administrators begin with all this? They start with good data. Without such data they cannot analyze situations, focus resources, or direct activities. The importance of good clinical/financial data is not Medicare reimbursement (DRGs); it is planning, managing, and communicating with physicians. The problem with focusing on Medicare pricing is that it covers only a part of the total patient population, is changing constantly, and is of limited use. Hospitals must not use one payer's regulations for setting the direction of the whole institution.

Clinical/financial information also is the key to bringing the physicians back into the management team. Case-mix type reports facilitate communication with medical staff members. After all, these are their data that managers are using. To develop the data base, administrators must:

- determine what data are needed and what are available
- develop a real data dictionary
- begin saving the available elements that are needed

- start accumulating the missing elements
- purify and improve the data collected.

The medical records department has become a significant party in the development of a good clinical/financial data base.

The next step is to develop the program analysis capability. This is an integral part of producing a good operating plan and a sound budget. Managers must look for a proved system that has broader analysis capabilities than do DRGs. Large hospitals, in particular, should seek a system that can capture and analyze data at a detailed procedure level. Procedure data should be collected as of the date of service and the computer system should be able to associate that information with a patient in a given hospital room. This capability will be extremely important because it will be necessary to analyze nursing efforts as they relate to a particular patient on a particular day and to specific procedures. The system must be able to relate specific procedures prescribed to an expected order pattern for that specific patient group (a practice profile). The system also must be able to manipulate the costs for each procedure as well as the charges and the statistics.

The system must be flexible. That means it must be able to do many types of analysis, not just a few standard reports. Interestingly enough, all the software tools are available, and at varying price levels. For very little expense, an institution may receive a simple comparison of its cost per DRG with the Medicare prospective rates. For $25,000 and up, the hospital could receive an annual service on a shared basis, possibly with another institution or another hospital. For $75,000 to $85,000, the institution could install a complete dedicated minicomputer case-mix analysis system. For $80,000 to $90,000 management could obtain the software for a complete in-house mainframe supersystem.

Some of the new systems can manipulate procedure costs. At least actual order patterns can be compared with expected order patterns (practice profiles). Another system can utilize presenting problems and test results to group patients for analyzing expected treatment. Of course, there is always the possibility of developing a new custom system from scratch, which has no upper limit on cost. The considerations when dealing with clinical/financial data base information are the data quality, dependability, understandability, availability, flexibility of analysis, cost, and timeliness.

Time is a major consideration. Hospital administrators cannot wait to begin collecting the data and implementing a system. It will take two years or more just to produce quality analysis. As noted, the available data generally are not the quality most people think they are. Furthermore, several payers already have collected data about individual institutions and have built profiles. One payer has developed practice profiles for selected clinical patient groups. Those who focus on the changes brought about by Medicare prospective payment fail to recognize the impact of the methods being instituted by almost all payers.

DEPARTMENTAL RESPONSIBILITIES

Physicians

There is a certain amount of manager frustration when physicians do not participate actively in hospital management. Physicians have strong political positions in medical centers and community hospitals and sometimes use this status to comment on the management process without participating in it and without accepting responsibility for results. Sometimes they sit back and critique "administration" decisions and separate themselves from "administration" when it is convenient.

The use of a program orientation for managing the hospital requires the participation of physicians. They must help analyze the data, define programs, identify resource requirements, and develop management systems that link actual results to long-term goals. They also must participate in the budget process. The budget is a control tool. It supplies the comparison of measurable actual results to a specific measurable goal. Because goals are program based, the budget must be as well. Physicians are responsible for programs (for example, rehabilitation, normal deliveries, or open-heart surgery), so they must take active roles in the budget process.

To make the budget process effective, managers must provide physicians with analyses showing volume and other statistics by specialty and subspecialty. Physicians (department heads) must be asked to forecast patient days, admissions, lengths of stay, and resource utilization by specialty, subspecialty, specific physician group, or diagnostic program. They must review resource utilization, by program, and comment on variances in actual resource utilization by different physicians or groups from the expected utilization for the same program type of patient.

Physicians must play much more important roles in helping administrators understand the nature of patient requirements. In the past managers all too often relied upon the nursing workload index system to determine the appropriate staffing for nursing. Traditionally, those systems showed that patients constantly were becoming sicker and sicker, so nursing staff had to be increased. In the future, managers must use clinical/financial information in a matrix format to identify specific physicians who are utilizing the resources of a particular nursing unit. This kind of tool will allow management to go directly to the individual physicians and discuss the nature of the patients to ascertain whether, in fact, the patients next year will require more resources or a different type of service than those in the current year. This kind of information will prove much more informative to management in the budget process.

The budget obviously is a tool for communicating predictions of the future and allocating resources and, as noted, also is a tool for measuring actual activity against stated objectives. The implication is that just as a physician or group of doctors is required to participate in the development of the budget, those same individuals must be responsible for seeing that the budget goals are achieved.

Nursing

Nurses may well become the coordinators of program management. They carry out the physicians' orders and have significant input into patient care plans. Proper use of a clinical/financial data base should include broader involvement of the nursing staff. Nurses should be asked to participate in the analysis of the various types of patients and how they are being served (analyzing all the resource utilization). They also are a key element of the changes being made because, as noted, they represent 16 to 19 percent of the institution costs. In the past, administration did not measure nursing cost very well nor analyze it appropriately. Managers should ask nursing to establish standards based upon the number of minutes of nursing care required for each patient in the unit each day. By matching this information with the clinical/financial data for that particular patient, managers can better analyze and predict the nursing requirements for various types of patients. Hospitals have yet to understand how nursing costs vary throughout the stay of a particular patient or to find the patient characteristics that allow prospective determination of those nursing requirements. Institutions also have not communicated to payers and the consumer public how nursing requirements vary patient by patient.

Data Processing

At a recent social gathering someone said that if we had improved airplanes as much as we have improved computers over the last few years, we should be able to fly around the world in half an hour using no more than five gallons of fuel. Data processing technologies are developing faster than they can be utilized effectively.

As new systems are added, customers must turn toward those that are truly user oriented—those that are designed for users and can be operated primarily by them. This will take some of the pressure off hospitals' data processing shops. Administrators all too often have expected the data units to know everything about everything the managers do, to be able to read the executives' minds, and to be able to interpret their very vague desires into a specific set of instructions for the computers. It hasn't worked all that well.

Finance

Financial people must become planners. Their utility to the institution as accountants and number shufflers is decreasing. Technology has passed them by in many cases. Computer programs are doing much of the numbers crunching that accountants used to do, and much faster. Financial people also have to become better communicators. In many institutions, the financial staff remained closeted on the top floor in an old building next door to the hospital, or in the basement.

These groups must be brought out of their hiding place and begin working directly with the physicians, nurses, technicians, and administrators. They must begin sharing more of the data that they have kept so closely guarded for these many years and must begin helping the other groups to understand the materials.

Medical Records

Medical records personnel control the most important, least understood, and possibly most underutilized numbers in the data base. They have a leadership role in a number of areas but appear to be rather slow in adapting to their new responsibilities. They must help managers develop a quality data base that is accessible, dependable, and timely, as well as standards for evaluating the data and their accumulation. They also must educate administrators as to what the data mean.

In the near term, quality data relate directly to government payment. Hospitals must be extremely careful in how they report clinical data in order to make sure that they are being paid properly for the services they provide to Medicare recipients. Table 2–3 presents some interesting cases.

It is clear that the absence of quality data will mean no government payment. Quality data mean abstracting from full medical records (not just from the face

Table 2–3 Payment Rate Varies with Clinical Description

DRG	Description	U.S. Payment Rate per Case	Mean Length of Stay (Days)
438	Alcoholism w/Cirrhosis	$2,977	6.9
202	Cirrhosis w/Alcoholism	$4,230	9.3
32	Concussion	$1,598	3.3
25	Postconcussion Syndrome	$2,260	4.9
134	Hypertension w/Congestive Heart Failure	$2,492	6.1
127	Congestive Heart Failure w/Hypertension	$3,680	7.8

sheet); this means finding complications and comorbidities and bringing them into the first few secondary diagnoses (highlighting them in order to receive proper government payment). Quality data from an accountant's standpoint also mean consistency. This means reabstracting studies and audits to verify accuracy. Quality data mean making sure the right information makes its way to the hospital bill. Quality also means collection of data not required by the government, such as primary diagnoses.

The information accumulated by medical records must be ready for timely entry on the hospital bill. The bill cannot wait, because of cash-flow considerations. Management should be able to accumulate data within the normal four-day billing hold period.

Clinical information must be accessible. Management must be able to get its hands on a volume of recent data in a short time, which means intelligent use of computers. The information must be accurate and it must be available. In order to determine the quality of the material and its timeliness, accessibility, and dependability, managers need standards by which to evaluate the information.

Managers also need to know what the data say and what they mean, and who is better able than the medical records personnel to provide the education. That education should be at a management level and be part of the overall education process. Medical records staff members need to know why managers are asking them very specific questions, how they are using the data, and why they are in a hurry. Medical records then needs to help managers analyze the results of the studies using the data. Medical records also could play a role in the development of some of the new tools such as the ability to project resource utilization for a given patient's stay.

Medical records persons definitely must be part of the team to help managers develop the prospective criteria and possibly new measures for determining nursing staff requirements. They also must be part of the team that helps identify the trends management will need to anticipate future demands and their specific types.

THE IMPACT OF THE COST CUTS

The federal government is imposing constraints on health care costs and other payers are consolidating and cutting back. There will be reduced utilization, leading to consolidation of hospital industry resources. Over the longer term there will be fewer acute care hospital beds. There will be changes in the roles of many institutions and major alterations in the nature of others.

Administrators know what needs to be done:

- improve the management process and management tools
- start or improve data collection, education, and the development of manageable entities (programs)

- involve the physicians who will have direct responsibility for program management, programs being the focal point for planning and controlling the institution.

All of these changes must take place in a relatively short time because for the most part hospitals are behind and have to catch up. Any successful endeavor as large as this must be done on a step-by-step basis, with each step being completed successfully before the next one is begun.

Finally, the total change will have to take place "on the cheap." Managers cannot expect new resources coming from other areas to finance the development of new tools. The institution must generate the financing for those new tools by focusing its resources away from underutilized, undesirable, unprofitable programs. Recent changes, and others yet to come, will provide major challenges for hospital management. It will be interesting to see how many managers are able to develop more or better outcomes with decreasing demand.

NOTES

1. *Hospital Statistics*, 1984 ed. (Chicago: American Hospital Association, 1984), p. 7.

2. Maureen Metz, "Trends in Sources of Capital in the Hospital Industry," in *Report of the Special Committee on Equity of Payment for Not-for-Profit and Investor-Owned Hospitals* (Chicago: American Hospital Association, 1983).

3. Ibid.

4. William O. Cleverley, *The Hospital Industry Analysis Report 1981* (Healthcare Financial Management Association, 1982).

5. Ibid.

6. Paul B. Ginsburg and Malcolm J. Curtis, "Prospects for Medicare's Hospital Insurance Trust Fund," *Health Affairs* (Spring 1983): 102–11.

7. *Directions in Healthcare 1985–1987* (Healthcare Financial Management Association, 1985).

8. Ginsburg and Curtis, "Prospects."

9. Donald E.L. Johnson, "Buyer Picky in Growing Market," *Modern Health Care* 12, no. 5 (May 1982): 86–93.

Chapter 3

Organizational Structure and Management

David B. Starkweather

THE FEDERAL POLICY CONTEXT

Hospital considerations of integrated clinical and financial systems can well be seen in the larger context of changing national policies and health economics.

In 1982 and early 1983, at the federal level, there had arisen a fundamental and pervasive concern for the size of the national budget. That concern continues to this day; indeed, it has become greater. Since health care is a major component of the budget and since portions of that component are discretionary, it was natural that both the congressional and executive branches would focus on new methods of controlling such expenditures. A parallel concern involved the Medicare Trust Fund and the Social Security Fund. The projections were that the Trust Fund would be bankrupt by 1990 under terms of the existing provider reimbursement policies that had been called open-ended entitlement.

Another policy trend was more general and fundamental. The economic philosophies of Reaganomics were a marked departure from those of the preceding Carter administration. Administrators are familiar with the basic principles of this new philosophy as it applies to the health field:

1. a return to more competitive approaches, emphasizing vigorous markets
2. deregulation, particularly of prices
3. consumer participation in health care expenditures through increasing the proportion of patient co-payments, reducing the market-buffering effects of health insurance, and placing caps on the amount of employee tax-free health insurance premiums.

Related to this new posture was the accumulated history of federal government initiative and private activity concerning health maintenance organizations (HMOs). While HMOs did not take off at the pace early policy designers

33

envisioned, certainly their experience showed that the utilization of hospital and doctor services could be reduced substantially without apparent effect on quality. The Reagan Administration pulled back from continued funding of HMO development, but it did so with the realization that the concept had caught on with the business community and that there was every likelihood that the private dynamics of large businesses as purchasers of medical care would continue to expand this form of service delivery.

HMOs were only one interest of organized business, which by the early 1980s had come to recognize the tremendous costs of health insurance as a fringe benefit and which had changed its posture from passive acceptance of this condition to one of aggressive marketplace negotiation and enterprise. Many new approaches to the control of health care costs have developed from the private industrial sector, including preferred provider organizations (PPOs). In an effort to control fringe benefit costs, many employers no longer pay full premium costs for whatever health insurance their employees choose; they only will pay the HMO rate. This has left employee families with a choice of paying large percentages of premium costs themselves or switching their coverage to the various HMO options that work through controlling medical care utilization.

In short, the Reagan Administration's intent to activate private medical markets was beginning to work, at least insofar as participation of business and labor was concerned.

Federal policy changed in yet another respect as a result of the history of the health planning movement. The federal initiative had started in the early 1950s with grants to voluntary health planning agencies, had continued in 1965 with the funding and mandating of Comprehensive Health Planning Agencies, and had continued in 1975 through blanketing the nation with Health Systems Agencies. All of this appeared to have done little to control the costs of medical care. This was true even in areas of capital investments and expensive technologies where these regulatory agencies presumably had maximum clout. Study after study documented the failure of this form of franchising and regulation. These conclusions lent support to the critics of government regulation as a form of social and institutional control of hospitals.

Clearly, something new was needed if health care costs, both those incurred by the federal government and those of other parties, were to be brought under control. Federal policymakers concluded that the method of payment was at the root of this problem: cost reimbursement to hospitals and fee-for-service reimbursement to physicians.

These circumstances were expected to get worse under conditions of a surfeit rather than a shortage of doctors. Would not more doctors simply provide more services and order more tests as a means of livelihood, thus expanding even further the amount of expenditures? With payments to hospitals out of control under the terms of "reasonable cost" reimbursement, what would government payments be under fee-for-service reimbursement to an oversupply of physicians?

These, then, were the several forces that signaled some fundamental changes in federal law and in many state laws, combined with a different and more aggressive posture on the part of large-scale purchasers of health care through insurance. The changes were dramatic and came swiftly, because the conclusions were so fundamental:

1. Retrospective payment had to be elminated. There was simply no way marketplace incentives and penalties could be introduced into a system driven on historically defined costs.
2. Cost reimbursement for hospitals must be eliminated. While providers and government argued incessantly over what was "reasonable" and what should be a definable cost, the fundamental fact was that the existing reimbursement system was cost inducing. Again, there was no place for market forces to operate if greater revenues could be obtained simply by adding more services.
3. The focus should be on utilization of hospital services rather than on the unit cost of patient days. The experience with HMOs had demonstrated that control of utilization was possible and that indeed total hospital costs could be influenced much more dramatically by this intervention than by small variations in the definitions of reasonable cost or by trying to make certificate of need more effective.
4. Economic risk must be shifted from third parties to providers. As long as government and insurance companies carried the risk for health care costs, there was no incentive for providers to be concerned with such matters. Indeed, their concern was just the opposite: to maximize revenue through "creative accounting" on the part of hospitals and through "creative service definition" on the part of physicians.

THE DRG RESPONSE

Perhaps because of the swiftness of their action, federal policymakers adopted diagnosis related groups (DRGs) in ignorance of their total effects. These then unknown effects have had a good deal to do with the organizational and management implications and development.

One question is whether the new reimbursement system, with its strong emphasis on incentives and penalties, will work if it applies only to Medicare patients and not to all other payer classes. At the institutional level this payer mix creates an organizational nightmare. A typical hospital must deal with customers who pay on the basis of (1) capitation, (2) diagnostic category, (3) prices set by the hospital, (4) prices negotiated with bulk purchasers, (5) historically determined full cost, and (6) historically determined partial cost.

This induces nightmares for hospital managers because these six classes not only differ in their means of payment and collection but they set up motivations for organizational performance that conflict with one another. For instance, elements of an organization that are maximizing revenue under terms of a private or government historical cost reimbursement would be behaving poorly by standards established for those elements that are maximizing revenue on capitated or prospectively determined payments. Incentives and controls established for the medical and financial management of one class of patients are literally reversed for another class but doctors, nurses, and other hospital employees cannot discern such changes and shift their operations so quickly and frequently.

Another concern is whether the DRG system encourages low cost behavior based on reducing lengths of stay while at the same time encouraging higher admission rates, particularly for categories in which a hospital believes it can make money. If the overall strategy is to control costs through utilization, the system's incentives and penalties operate on only one of the two factors that determine utilization.

A third concern involves what has become known in the vernacular as "DRG creep," reclassifying patients' diagnoses in order to obtain more reimbursement. Simborg documents the opportunities, both ethical and unethical, for tinkering with the protocols and criteria for case-mix reimbursement in order to maximize revenue.[1] There should be no doubt that this will take place. After all, it is a natural institutional motivation, and it is known how successfully it was done by hospitals following the 1965 legislation when reimbursements were determined by the ratio of costs to charges. There already is a plethora of consultants and experts to help hospitals maximize their DRG-based reimbursements.

A fourth problem is the great heterogeneity of DRG groups. As discussed in Chapter 4 by Joseph S. Gonnella and Carter Zeleznik, the DRG system is insensitive to variations in severity of illness within groups. The system also is unstable with respect to changes in clinical practice. DRG reimbursement depends on entirely accurate and complete discharge codes. The true diagnoses and conditions of patients can be misrepresented, particularly for DRGs that have low articulation with respect to diagnosis.

Beyond the management of individual hospitals, another question is what the DRG system will do, or not do, for public hospitals, teaching hospitals, and other institutions that serve the poor and the more severely ill. Motivations stemming from DRGs are clear: eliminate services that are costlier to provide, or eliminate categories of patients whose service is costlier. Where will patients in these categories go and what is the destiny of the institutions that serve them primarily?

In sum, there was little consideration for how the DRG system, with its expenditure limits and its new incentives and penalties, would alter institutional decision making and the hospital system. Some of the unintended consequences that have been generated by this system of reimbursement rewards and penalties are emerging.

Medicare-sponsored patients are only one payer class for most community hospitals; there is an analogous set of cross-cutting incentives and penalties for nongovernment patients. Any number of contracts with PPOs may have been struck for services that are discounted from a hospital's full charges. These prices assume the hospital can operate above its marginal costs, albeit below full average costs. Yet such operational targets and motivations are different from those associated with full cost reimbursement established on a historical basis. Here, fixed cost behavior is to be maximized because it will be reimbursed, leading to greater revenues.

There is the case of hospitals serving patients enrolled in capitated prepaid health plans. If the health plan that is sponsoring patients is an external purchaser of care, the hospital is interested in increasing the volume of inpatients, assuming the price negotiated for their care is above marginal costs. But if the hospital is itself an owner of the health plan, perhaps in conjunction with its doctors, then reduced rather than increased volumes of hospitalization are desired, since the plan will produce more money from the difference between actual and anticipated utilization. Again, the managerial and operational motivations are conflicting, yet all are operating within the same organization. The pathway to a decent bottom line is indeed varied.

This, then, is the larger context in which new clinical and financial hospital control systems must be seen. Specifically, these changes in the policy and economic environment require integration of clinical and financial elements not only in hospital systems but also in management structures. In recent decades there has developed a separation of these functions in most U.S. hospitals, primarily because nonphysicians have assumed so much of administration. Now these functions must be integrated in new, decentralized organization structures. This is because the new imperatives call for joint management of these functions in order to control hospital utilization of all kinds, to obtain a new service or product line emphasis, and to become more efficient under strong market and competitive forces.

Four realms of consideration relate directly to hospital organization and management:

1. changes in administrative structures and functions
2. changes in the organization of hospital medical practice and medical staffs

3. changes in the relationships among medical staff, management, and governance
4. changes in industry structure.

CHANGES IN ADMINISTRATION

Case-mix reimbursement provides a new impetus or justification for strategic planning. This is because an analysis of programs and services by case mix will beg the questions of whether hospitals should take on services that attract winning DRGs and drop services that are losers.

Another important aspect of strategic planning and financial analysis is the consideration of new and expensive technologies. Since case-mix reimbursement may not cover certain such technologies, and since even traditional ones are being used in different ways and with reduced volume, the strategic planning process is being altered.

A third newly emphasized activity is the medical records function. At least two aspects of medical records are changing dramatically and increasing in importance: (1) the medical record as an accurate clinical document, and (2) the medical record as an input to a medical management information system. Only the first of these is discussed here since the second is examined in Chapter 1. Only organizational and management ramifications are dealt with here.

Hospitals must have the professional and technical capacity to have every medical record completed upon discharge. In fact, much has to be completed while patients are in the hospital. Part of this imperative is a function of medical records administration and part involves the medical staff. Hospital employees must perform concurrent DRG analysis based on preliminary diagnoses provided by admitting physicians. This constitutes an early warning mechanism in respect to physician treatment patterns.

As to which kind of persons are best suited to perform this function, the possibilities are: medical records personnel, nurses, finance personnel, physicians, or a new type of employee trained specifically for this activity. The author regards medical records personnel as the most appropriate. If this is the choice, such persons must become knowledgeable of the financial implications of DRG reimbursement.

The technical job of diagnostic classification should be separated from the follow-on task involving what is done with the results of these classifications. The concern here is further analysis of patient diagnosis and care, education and discipline of practitioners, and the host of activities that provide future hospital medical practice with strong components of finance and economics. While a variety of people will become involved in this stream of activities, at this point the role of nurses should be mentioned. Nurses are in positions to identify and monitor consumption patterns by diagnostic category and by doctor. They are in positions to make the process concurrent rather than historical. Just as nurses have become important in utilization control, so are they important in case-mix control. Administration can expect an expanded role for nurses in this regard and a need for their broadened education in finance, information systems, and general management.

As for management structure, it has been shown that hospitals as organizations face greater problems with a mix of patients under different reimbursement modes—DRG, capitation, cost, and price—than if the care of all patients were reimbursed in the same manner. A major challenge to hospital management is to set up structures that allow effective performance and optimization for each of these categories while not creating systems that are either so complicated or operate at such internal cross-purposes that everything is ineffective.

In general, case-mix reimbursement should move hospitals toward case-mix management, which means product management. Product management can take several forms, all of them variations of matrix management, in which a structure that identifies different products or services such as categories of DRGs is added to the traditional management structure that emphasizes functions. Table 3–1 illustrates this concept. The columns represent the typical organization of hospitals by function: activities that are similar are grouped together and each group is placed under the responsibility and authority of a hospital manager. The rows represent products or service lines of the hospital: groupings of patients with similar diagnosis or treatment patterns. As an example one hospital known to the author defined the following seven case-mix groupings: (I) medical-surgical; (II) cardiovascular; (III) oncology; (IV) mental health; (V) respiratory; (VI) women and infants; and (VII) orthopedic-neurologic-rehabilitation. In matrix management the operating employees of the hospital, whose jobs are allocated to the various cells of the matrix, have responsibilities both to the appropriate functional manager and to the appropriate product manager.

Table 3–1 Hospital Matrix Management

		Hospital Functions		
Hospital Products	*Finance*	*Professional Services*	*Patient Care Activities*	*Institutional Support Services*
Case-Mix Grouping I				
Case-Mix Grouping II				
Case-Mix Grouping III				
Case-Mix Grouping IV				
Case-Mix Grouping V				
Case-Mix Grouping VI				
Case-Mix Grouping VII				

Another hospital system known to the author initiated a product line approach to strategic planning, using a form of portfolio analysis derived from business and industry. First, it analyzed its own operations, those of its competitor hospitals, and that of the community or market, all through data obtained from its own operation, its local health systems agency, and a state agency that mandated reporting of hospital utilization and financial data. Diagnosis related categorization revealed several clusters that could be called product, service, or business lines:

ob/gyn/neonatology	rehabilitation
psychiatry	oncology/hematology
substance abuse	renal/male reproductive
cardiology/circulatory/	general surgery
respiratory	plastic/skin/burn
digestive/metabolic	eye/ear/dental
neurosciences/musculoskeletal	infectious diseases

Each of these service lines was then carefully assessed on three dimensions (a modification of the usual two-dimensional evaluation common in portfolio analysis). Each line was evaluated in respect to (1) present and potential strength if a two-hospital system is the provider, (2) the attractiveness of the service line in the market, and (3) the community need for the service. Criteria were developed and applied for each of these dimensions, typically numbering eight or ten for each of the three.

From this, the strategic plan was developed, complete with long- and short-range tactics for expansion or shrinkage of service lines, priorities for the allocation of budgeted funds, and the assignment of opportunities for venture capital from the hospital system's strategic investment fund.

Another hospital system known to the author has turned the service line approach to its management structure. For each of its service lines it identified product managers. At first each service line had a group of managers operating partly as a coordinating committee and partly as a management team. This proved too cumbersome and lacked effectiveness so the teams were replaced with a single manager with clearly defined authority.

In any matrix system of management there must be a careful allocation of authority and power between service or product managers and functionally oriented managers. Conflict between these two types can be expected. In this instance the conflict was accentuated initially by the fact that in a system involving three merged hospitals, even with the three institutions in close proximity, the functional managers retained their former hospital orientations while the product managers adapted the new systemwide orientation. This strain, caused in part by the newness of the three-hospital merger, has since subsided.

It can be concluded from this that a matrix type of service line management would be easier to install in a stand-alone hospital. Yet it also can be concluded that if hospitals are in a system that spans facilities providing services to a common market, then a systemwide matrix is the sensible way to restructure.

A variation on this is a matrix that has a service line makeup relating to case-mix groups and also incorporates a hospital's geographic or physical areas, thus allowing product management through the relocation and reassignment of several types of personnel such as medical records and financial.

Under either type there must be product managers. Who should these persons be? One hospital has identified physicians for these positions. Another has assigned nurses through redefinition of the traditional head nurse role. In still another, certain department heads function in this capacity.[2] And a fourth has positioned its assistant administrators in these roles. In all instances, these persons must be capable of spanning both clinical and financial orientations.

There are both rewards and penalties in case-mix and prospective reimbursement that hospitals are not used to. Hospitals can be more entrepreneurial in their operations. If they stand to benefit or lose financially by these reimbursement methods, they should pass these potentials on to their service line managers, as well as to others. These forms of reimbursement require a new focus on hospital efficiency and effectiveness. It is important to capture and reward innovations that lead in these directions, so incentive pay schemes and joint ventures with product managers will become more common.

These changing management requirements have implications for university programs that educate persons for hospital administration, and for continuing management education. Hospitals can expect more graduates who have both clinical and financial backgrounds, more who are quantitatively and analytically prepared to tackle institutional efficiency and productivity, and more who are prepared for the assumption of business risk.

CHANGES IN MEDICAL STAFF ORGANIZATION

It has been said that "doctors are not in the system"—referring to hospital financial and operational matters as "the system." Case-mix reimbursement and service line management require that they do become involved. The dictum is that physicians must practice medicine by incorporating economic as well as clinical factors in their decision making.

One way to view this new focus is to draw attention to the normal and traditional medical staff functions that should receive new emphasis. This involves extending oversight activities relating to utilization review into the area of medical/financial audits undertaken on a concurrent basis. This process will not be as deliberate in its evolution as the prior procedures to which physicians were accustomed. For example, in past years the development of medical audits typically involved, in sequence: (1) participation by physicians in the development of criteria, (2) application of those criteria to the performance of medical practice, and (3) adjustment of some sort in either practicing behavior or the audit criteria. For the new medical/financial audits, statistical profiles are available immediately from clinical and management information systems and are presented to practicing physicians and their medical staff leaders for immediate action.

There will be a relentless process of monitoring, educating, and disciplining practitioners in respect to case-mix performance—a job initiated or accomplished by service line management. Exactly what mix of control strategies will result will vary greatly by circumstance. Robert Ambrose, medical director of the Morristown (N.J.) Memorial Hospital, has identified seven causes of "negative variance" in case-mix management:[3]

1. inappropriate physician practice habits
2. avoidable scheduling delays
3. breakdowns in physician communication
4. severity of illness
5. social reasons that prevent hospital discharge
6. new technologies that are not reimbursed
7. new procedures that are not used.

Ambrose emphasizes that there are numerous reasons why there may be negative case-mix variance, only some of which relate directly to physician practice. He recommends that the organized effort to deal with variance be undertaken in a spirit of positive education rather than punitive discipline. Even so, there are physicians in New Jersey who have been "disassociated" from their hospital medical staffs because of their DRG behavior.

These several new activities have been presented as extensions of the normal functions of an open medical staff. However, they may lead in time to a restructured medical staff that is more closed than open. Within the traditional medical staff structure there can develop subgroups of doctors organized to practice corporately, with the hospital contracting or initiating joint ventures with them for certain functions in clinical/financial management. These subgroups could match the service line pattern of the hospital.

Physicians have grave concerns about certain aspects of hospital case-mix management and reimbursement. One is that they are left exposed to malpractice charges. This stems from legal precedent having to do with the community standard of care and how case-mix management, including the financial aspect of audits, may inhibit physicians from meeting that standard.

A related concern for physicians is the potential erosion of quality. It certainly is possible for the new system of incentives and penalties to drive hospital medical care to a subquality level. While the initial concern involved the elimination of overuse or inappropriate use, the problem in the future may well be the underuse that can lead to substandard care.

Physicians are concerned on behalf of their patients that the application of case-mix management for some individuals will cause hospitals to shift costs to other patients, resulting in inequitable charges. This is an old issue in hospital management and will not disappear until or unless there is an all-payer method of reimbursement. Short of that, the active intervention of the business community is likely to prevent excessive cost shifting or differential pricing through demands for negotiated rates for HMO and PPO patients that will yield the same hospital prices for non-Medicare patients as exist under case-mix reimbursement.

CHANGES IN THE TOP MANAGEMENT TRIANGLE

Modifications within the medical staff were the focus of the previous section; this one deals with changes among the major organizational elements of the hospital: management, medical staff, and trustees. Traditionally, the hospital has had to concern itself only with a narrow range of production that involved the transfer of input factors such as labor, supplies, and facilities into "intermediate products" such as days of nursing care, laboratory tests, medications, and meals. Physicians then took these intermediate products and produced a more final output of patients with diagnosis, treatment, or rehabilitation.

But case-mix reimbursement has expanded the scope of hospital production, requiring new relationships between the institution and its physicians in order to obtain a new effectiveness. DRGs relegate to the past a behavior in which the hospital could concentrate solely on its various intermediate activities and ignore the effects of these on final treatment outcomes. Physicians can no longer regard the hospital as a "workshop" where patients may be housed in order to get certain institutional services, while ignoring the effects of their diagnosis and treatment regimes on hospital operating and financial results. Thus there is a requirement for a new physician-hospital partnership.

How can this new physician-hospital integration be implemented? Already described are the development of service line and case-mix management structures and procedures. There are other approaches.

One is to designate a new hospital-based physician to bridge the gap. In New Jersey, physician/managers have come into use. These persons, called variously medical director or vice president for medical affairs, have administrative authority within the hospital relating to effectiveness plus certain medical authority within the medical staff relating to treatment of patients. A similar development in a progressive California hospital is described by Aird and Skillicorn.[4] Essentially, these persons monitor and discipline the hospital on case-mix performance. Their backgrounds vary. They often are drawn from the ranks of the local medical staff. For the longer run, the education and development of such persons through formal training of physicians in management can be envisioned. Graduate programs in health services management are becoming populated with M.D.s.

Another mechanism is greater involvement of physicians in financial as well as strategic planning. This will serve the dual ends of introducing more clinical elements into hospital strategic decision making and educating physicians in the necessities of treating patients using financial criteria.

A new and closer working relationship between physicians and nurses can emerge as nurses become knowledgeable about the types and volume of hospital resources that physicians are consuming and are in a position to work with them as well as the various hospital support departments.

A change of great import stems from a combination of case-mix reimbursement and the movement toward HMOs and PPOs: the organization of physicians into new groups that take on responsibility of utilization control as a part of the assumption of actuarial risk for the cost of medical care to premium holders. These groups contract with hospitals for medical care that includes these control elements. The hospital-physician relationship will change from one represented entirely by the traditional medical staff organization, with physicians relating to the hospital on a one-by-one basis, to one in which the prime relationship for the hospital is with several medical groups, leaving the traditional staff organization for nongrouped physicians. This will be a source of tension, since these new groups will expect a direct role in hospital policy making, whereas such avenues traditionally have been through the medical staff structure with its elected service chiefs, executive body, and officers.

Hospital trustees can be expected, individually and collectively, to exercise more responsibility in medical staff credentialling, medical audits, and physicians' performance in relationship to case-mix reimbursement. It has been said that case-mix and prospective reimbursement will finally "make hospital trustees behave like board members." This means that their knowledge of hospital affairs will increase, their decision making will become more focused and operationally oriented, and their commitment and involvement to the institution's goals and activities will become more strategic.

It follows that hospital managements and boards will be drawn into closer juxtaposition and that the points of contact for policy making and decision making between boards and medical staffs will increase. The need for medical expertise on boards will increase. The obligation for physicians so appointed will be greater than in the past to behave as corporation directors and not as representatives of the medical profession.

CHANGES IN THE MEDICAL DELIVERY SYSTEM

This element involves changes in the structure of the industry. It now is clear that the new emphasis on product effectiveness will yield shorter lengths of stay and, ultimately, reduced admission rates. This means that hospitals will shrink in size as inpatient institutions while at the same time the patients who are admitted will be more acutely ill. The incentives and penalties built into case-mix reimbursement will stimulate a greater focus on efficiency in the use of labor and supplies. There also will be an increase in the purchase and use of cost-reducing equipment and technology.

As the level of case-mix reimbursement lowers in relation to what reimbursement has been historically, hospitals will become much more competitive with each other, with cost-efficient institutions dominating and those unable or unwilling to be efficient going under. This process will be heightened by the activities of business and industry as purchasers who will price shop by looking at costs and rates across hospitals and targeting certain institutions for negotiation and contract.

Hospital survival will be related not only to general operating efficiency but also to greater attention to the particular services provided. The importance of strategic planning has been discussed. This includes the development of services and the recruitment of patients in some service categories, while reducing services and discouraging patients in others. This is a fundamental change in the goals and operation of many community hospitals, most of which traditionally have seen themselves as providers of all services needed and serving patients of all economic levels.

Two aspects of this fundamental change will lead to industry restructuring:

1. Patients who are more severely ill will tend to be admitted or transferred to teaching and public hospitals, which will become burdened with high-cost patients who are difficult to serve and for which DRG-related reimbursement is insufficient. An increase also can be expected in investor-owned hospitals that will move fast in the marketplace to attract patients with low severity and high reimbursement categories—again leaving the burden for the treatment of difficult patients to others.
2. Hospitals will specialize in particular service lines or diagnostic groupings. The idea that the "general hospital has a general responsibility" will diminish in favor of a degree of specialization across hospitals by service lines. This cross-specialization will require new structures for trade-offs between institutions. On the one hand, free-standing hospitals will be cooperating and collaborating to the extent of determining which services are provided by which hospitals without duplications while on the other hand they will be competing aggressively. They also may simply compete fiercely and let the hidden hand of the marketplace make these allocations. Many hospital managers regard this as unworkable behavior but it will bring the hospital business closer to what is naturally the case in other business sectors.

Research completed in 1986 by the author shows that in highly competitive hospital markets yet another pattern of restructuring takes place.[5] As recently as 1982 in a highly competitive metropolitan community there were 12 free-standing community, religious, and government hospitals. By 1985 there were essentially four hospital systems, with the 12 previously independent hospitals having merged or affiliated into (1) a county hospital/medical school combine, (2) a three-facility community hospital system; (3) an HMO system embracing two hospitals, and (4) pending agreements on a religious hospital system embracing three previously separate hospitals.

In the process most competitors had changed into varying combinations of system alliances, and the level and type of competition had shifted from one based on service-by-service competition to a struggle for market shares that are sufficiently broad geographically for the systems to compete for patients sponsored by capitation-based prepaid health plans. The allocation of service lines among the hospitals had shifted from one previously based on certificate-of-need type regulation to the duplications of the open marketplace, and now finally to the internal decision making of the hospital systems as corporations.

In short, horizontal integration has completely restructured this hospital market, with rationalization of service lines across the community being accomplished primarily by new parent corporations of the merged or affiliated hospitals, a process and a result quite different from the situation that would have existed if the numerous original hospitals had remained independent competitors.

Just as individual hospitals will structure new horizontal relationships with each other, so will they also pursue new vertical relationships. Thus, hospitals will increase preadmission and postdischarge services as tests and procedures are shifted to outpatient bases and as facilities develop more comprehensive preadmission and postdischarge services as both a cause and an effect of reduced inpatient use.

A marked increase can be expected in diversification activities. Again, new structures will be needed to accomplish vertical integration for those instances where it is achieved through interorganization links rather than through internal development. New forms of joint ventures between hospitals and physician groups will emerge as each recognizes the need for the other in this kind of development. These arrangements will be true business joint ventures, with each party contributing developmental funds and each sharing in risks and returns.

THE OVERALL OUTLOOK

In sum, the specifics of case-mix reimbursement will change; procedural tinkering is inevitable. But the basic reforms in the financing of hospital care will not. These are prospective reimbursement based on price and the reassignment of risk from payers to providers.

Hospital decision making at the operations level will be altered to integrate clinical and administrative factors and to speed up decision making with effective information systems. Long-run and strategic planning will receive new emphasis, with greater focus on program and service mix. Organizational structures will become more product/management oriented, with a commensurate stress on both market-oriented product line development and institutionally oriented efficiency in hospital operations and medical practice.

Medical staffs will move toward policies and procedures that reflect the heavy impact of physician practice on hospital economics. Medical staffing, credentialling, education, discipline, and control all will be undertaken with new urgency. More fundamentally, the traditional role of the medical staff as the conduit for doctor-hospital relations may recede in favor of new contractual or joint venture relationships between physician groups and the hospital, based on negotiated self-interests.

Finally, relationships between health care organizations will change as hospitals compete, on the one hand using mixed strategies of vertical integration through diversification, and on the other hand horizontal relations at least sufficient to reallocate services. Both vertical and horizontal integrations will require new corporate forms, often of an entrepreneurial nature.

All of this will (and should) beg some fundamental questions of hospitals: Why are they in operation? Who really are the clients? Who is it important to serve? What do they stand for?

NOTES

1. D.W. Simborg, "Sounding Board: DRG Creep," *New England Journal of Medicine* 304 (June 25, 1981): 1602–4.
2. R.G. Goodrich and G.R. Hastings, "St. Luke's Hospital Reaps Benefits by Using Product Line Management," *Modern Healthcare* 15 (February 15, 1985).
3. R.M. Ambrose, unpublished manuscript, July 1984.
4. J.A. Aird and S.L. Skillicorn, "Innovative Structures for Medical Staff Organization," *Frontiers of Health Services Management* (February 1985).
5. D.B. Starkweather and J.M. Carman, "Horizontal and Vertical Concentrations in the Evolution of Hospital Competition," in R.M. Scheffler and L.F. Rossiter, eds. *Advances in Health Economics and Health Services Research*, Vol. 7. Greenwich, CT: JAI Press. (In press).

Chapter 4

Prospective Reimbursement Using the DRG Case-Mix Classification System: A Medical Perspective

Joseph S. Gonnella and *Carter Zeleznik*

The interest in medical case-mix classification arises out of increasing costs of health care and the introduction of the prospective reimbursement system by Medicare and Medicaid payers. A prospective reimbursement system of health care payment could be based upon an infinite number of different disease classification systems or on considerations unrelated to individuals' health and illness altogether.

In the prior retrospective system, payment was made on the basis of charges incurred in the treatment of a patient, with the only proviso being that the charges be "reasonable" in relation to the individual's needs. This approach was felt to be unworkable, however, because it appeared to encourage health care providers to order tests and other procedures that patients might not have needed. Policing of what patients needed in comparison with what they received proved to be difficult and relatively ineffective. There always seemed to be some mitigating circumstances for any procedure being ordered, no matter how outrageous it might appear when examined after the fact.

Detailed chart review to identify inappropriate provider decisions also proved not to be an attractive activity for professionals, and other individuals were thought to be unprepared to review clinical decisions.

NEED FOR DISEASE CLASSIFICATION

For a prospective reimbursement system to work, a disease classification procedure was needed. Selection of an appropriate procedure had to be based upon multiple criteria and take into account many considerations. Obviously, reimbursement based on the patient's weight would be frivolous and on age alone would be arbitrary (although to some extent this has in fact been built into the system that was adopted). Clearly, attention must be directed to the criteria used in selection of the disease classification system that was accepted; this requires that attention also be directed to criteria that should have been used.

The criteria that ultimately were used in selecting the diagnosis related group (DRG) system included the following:

- The classification system should provide distinct clusters of patients. There should be no ambiguity with regard to which classification group a given patient would be assigned to.
- The classification system should take into account multiple interests of different groups of individuals including:

  1. society (third party payers, including the federal government and insurance companies)
  2. users of the system (i.e., patients and potential patients and their families)
  3. institutions that provide health care services (i.e., hospitals and clinics)
  4. physicians and other health care professionals.

- The classification should have some empirical foundations that demonstrate its practical feasibility (i.e., it should have been field tested); classification units should demonstrate certain statistical properties of interest, especially those of homogeneity with regard to the groupings that developed when patient data were examined.
- Classification categories should be limited—one million patients should not be put into one million different categories.

It clearly was not easy to meet these criteria. Indeed, it would appear that consideration was given to the criteria almost as an afterthought since the Congressional hearings on adopting the DRG system were conducted over a very short period and gave little attention to competing approaches. What clearly is lacking in the system as adopted is what may be called "medical meaningfulness." Homogeneity can be obtained in many ways. If different groups of patients are analyzed in terms of resources utilized, homogeneity may be found, but their health problems may have been quite different and some or much of the resource utilization may be inappropriate.

This chapter addresses some of the issues related to the criterion concerned with medical meaningfulness in case classification. The other criteria can best be served only when this condition is met as a prior consideration. To the extent that this has not occurred in designing and implementing the DRG approach, it may be expected that (1) health care delivery to numbers of patients will be compromised or that (2) the objective of reducing or controlling health care costs will not be met.

To understand concepts related to medical meaningfulness in disease classification, it is important to recognize the central role classification has played in the recent history of science. A century ago, the primary activity of scientists involved the classification of objects and of organisms in the natural world. The classification systems they developed concentrated on examining essential characteristics of these entities and on determining what constituted essential characteristics to begin with. In many cases, superficial appearances were recognized as misleading.

Problems of classification remain unsolved today even in the natural world. It is recognized now that no perfect system of classification exists or can be constructed. Classification is something that humans impose upon nature but does not exist as such in nature. Scientists in all fields recognize this. In order to classify, it is necessary to simplify. This means that certain data must be disregarded, and this in turn limits or distorts what is being classified.

In general, one goal of any system is to ensure that what is being classified is homogeneous within any category. In this regard, the purpose of the classification activity may be of paramount interest. In the medical area, it is reasonable to classify on the basis of similarities in disease conditions. This facilitates rational medical treatment of individuals who are ill. Of course, individual characteristics, including age and weight, also must be taken into account as well as factors such as the skills of providers and the availability of specific services. The thesis of this chapter, however, is that an optimal classification system in medicine allows individuals with "similar illnesses" to be treated in the same or similar ways. This would tend to ensure that outcomes would be similar and that costs would be similar as well.

The problem is how to define "similar illness" in practical terms. Even though there may be biological similarities among patients, there will be a number of factors that will affect what care they receive, as noted; their expectations and demands for care also will vary, which will influence the effectiveness of the treatment.

Case-mix classification thus is an exercise in how best to pretend that what is in fact heterogeneous is homogeneous. The real challenge is to reduce heterogeneity without promoting inappropriate homogeneity.

Specific questions that may be asked in this regard include:

- How can/should similarity in disease be defined? What are the essential characteristics of disease that allow different diseases to be classified in common categories?
- How much similarity, homogeneity, or specificity is needed for a given system of classification to be effective?
- When in the treatment process should definitions of similarity be applied: before, during, or after—or all of these?

• What other factors will or should influence the utilization of resources in the health care area?

PROSPECTIVE REIMBURSEMENT

As discussed, reimbursement for health care services in hospitals was on a retrospective basis until implementation of the two major Congressional bills: P.L. 97-248, the Tax Equity and Fiscal Responsibility Act of 1982 (TEFRA), which required prospective payment to hospitals, and P.L. 98-21, the Social Security Amendments of 1983, which shifted Medicare payments to hospitals to a prospective basis and established the DRG system. Under the prior system, upon patients' departure from the hospital, all charges were calculated and totaled. Some patients might have had very extensive and expensive workups. Others, with essentially the same health problems, might have been treated in different ways with lower charges. Many third party payers would pay on a per diem basis, with rates that might vary, depending upon volume.

The relation between charges and actual costs of providing hospital care generally would not be clearly established and might not even be known. This form of payment was similar to what is found in many situations, such as in getting a car repaired. Although there may be initial estimates of what is required to be done, final charges are a function of what actually was done.

It is generally believed that the retrospective reimbursement system did not work effectively and was responsible in large measure for steadily escalating health care costs. (Of course, it also may be argued that the system of payment is a secondary factor and that the primary issue involves physician and patient behaviors that to some extent are functions of the fact that payment for care is under the control of third party groups.)

In any event, the alternative approach endorsed by the federal government involves prospective reimbursement. This prospective payment system (PPS) does not mean that payment is made in advance for health care services that will be provided to patients in the future; rather, it means that payment will be made in the future on the basis of the patients' condition and the reason for hospitalization determined after hospitalization. Based upon the assignment made, a formula is applied that sets the exact amount of payment to be made, regardless of (1) what happens to the patient, (2) how long the patient stays, and (3) multiple considerations about the patient's condition that may affect these matters. A better word to describe these procedures might be "predetermined."

The prospective or predetermined reimbursement system was phased into the health care system beginning October 1, 1983, for patients seeking hospital health care services as part of the Medicare program of the Social Security system, with full implementation in 1986. This system provides for payment for care given to patients without regard to the specifics of what services are in fact provided, except for certain classification categories that take into account major surgical interventions. The key concept involves payments on the basis of average costs for various categories of illness, with those averages being computed on a national basis.

In principle, therefore, even though there might be considerable variation within a given category, payments are fixed and do not vary. The predetermined payment system allows the hospital to make a profit on patients who require or who receive, for whatever reason, fewer tests or less intensive care. Similarly, hospitals sustain losses on patients whose care involves greater demands on the system than the hypothetical average case within a given category. The hospital "wins" financially if a patient dies shortly after admission but "loses" if the person survives a relatively long hospitalization.

At issue, then, is to determine whether this classification system does effectively categorize patients into disease categories in a way that ensures equity with regard to their real needs and at the same time protects hospitals that care for individuals whose real needs may be greater and who thus place excessive demands on the institution's resources. Insofar as government reimbursement policies tend to lead the way for changes in procedures by other health care providers, the result has been major shifts in the entire system of payment since 1983. For example, in Philadelphia, the Blue Cross has announced a reimbursement system based upon average charges of patients at different hospitals. No differentiation is made for disease or the patient's condition and the only variable taken into consideration is the average charge of the hospital in which care is provided. All DRGs effectively become a single DRG that varies, however, from hospital to hospital. It is anticipated that these changes will greatly affect the practice of medicine and the health care that people receive. Issues of social justice are likely to come into play. In any event, multiple changes can be expected in how health care is provided in this country.

All this poses some major questions:

1. Is the status quo actually being maintained in spite of "cosmetic" changes?
2. At what point in an individual's hospital stay should the illness be classified for purposes of reimbursement?
3. Should illness be classified after medical or surgical intervention, as provided for by the PPS and DRG system?
4. How can "similar illness" be defined operationally?
5. How medically meaningful is the new disease classification system to physicians?
6. To what extent does the new system tend to reward the use of surgical procedures in patient care?
7. To what extent may costly special units with sophisticated technology and highly trained personnel be underutilized in efforts to reduce costs?

8. To what extent does the underutilization of such sophisticated units lead to high mortality or greater morbidity that might have been prevented?
9. To what extent will developmental work in high technology suffer from a reallocation of priorities or affect costs and other outcomes?
10. To what extent have hospitals developed policies that prevent or discourage their admitting very sick patients who require significant resources for optimal care?
11. To what extent are hospitals tempted to discharge patients prematurely and, if necessary, to readmit them at a later time, perhaps under a different disease classification?
12. To what extent is hospital specialization encouraged that may be desirable economically and may be good in terms of quality of care in certain areas but also may reduce the range of services that the facility offers to the community?
13. What types of conflicts among hospital administrators, nurses, and the medical staff are resulting from the changes?
14. How are decisions being made in hospitals so that both quality and cost control are addressed objectively?
15. To what extent has a need arisen for physicians and administrators to develop an internal management system that allows both parties to make economically sound decisions without disrupting the quality of care?
16. To what extent does the new reimbursement system penalize physicians who care for sicker patients, especially if the individuals are being treated medically rather than surgically?
17. To what extent are physicians whose patients' needs require greater resources being denied hospital privileges? What will be the legal consequences of this?

THE DEFINITION OF DISEASE

To classify anything, it is necessary to start with a general and valid definition of what it is that is being classified. Clearly, in the health care delivery system, disease classification for whatever purpose requires a definition of what a disease is. Distinctions then may be made among different diseases to permit medical diagnoses to be made and treatment to be effective. Indicators of diseases (i.e., disease symptoms or signs or, as they often are called, "problems") should not be confused with or thought to be equivalent to the diseases. If the indicators of disease are mixed with the diseases, confusion is likely to result. This is especially the case when it is realized that different diseases may have the same symptoms or signs.

Symptoms and signs have a static quality to them. However, diseases, regardless of their manifestations, are not static entities—they are dynamic processes. The disease processes may be slow or rapid in development. They may affect only selected parts (i.e., organs or organ systems) of an individual or they may result in death, which affects all organs.

Four criteria that should be used to define disease entities effectively are:[1]

1. There must be an identifiable etiological factor or set of factors that causes specific pathophysiological changes in the organism. Failure to specify such etiological agents indicates incomplete disease identification. (Of course, the etiological agents associated with certain "diseases" are unknown, which makes it necessary to work with an incomplete definition in those cases.)
2. There must be a specific organ or organs affected by the etiological agent. A common error in medical diagnosis is to identify an organ in which some malfunction or structural change has occurred that is indicative of disease but in which the responsible etiological agent is not identified. Such an incomplete diagnosis may be classified as a health problem. Health problems such as congestive heart failure (CHF) may affect many body systems, but without additional information the disease entity responsible for this condition cannot be known. (Merely to assert that the organism is under attack by a particular etiological agent such as a virus without specifying what organ or organ system of the body is involved is also an inadequate definition of disease.)
3. There must be some characteristic pathophysiological changes in the organ or organ system involved. These changes are the clinical signs or symptoms mentioned above. For example, peptic ulcer is likely to have as an associated or secondary characteristic upper gastrointestinal bleeding, but such bleeding may occur in response to other disease conditions as well.
4. The severity of the pathophysiological changes must be determined relative to the disease process as an evolving, dynamic entity. This can be done most easily through specification of what is called "disease stage." Diabetes mellitus, like other disease entities, must be thought of in terms of a sequence of pathophysiological changes including hyperglycemia, diabetic acidosis, diabetic retinopathy, peripheral neuropathy, and azotemia secondary to renal damage. These changes may be further defined as well, so the extent of hyperglycemia, acidosis, retinopathy, neuropathy, or azotemia must be specified in order for a diagnosis to be made and the disease to be defined adequately. Similarly, pneumococcal pneumonia with septicemia is a different disease from pneumococcal pneumonia complicated by either empyema or meningitis. Failure to classify disease in terms of severity or stage is probably the most common deficiency found in medical diagnoses and in medical records. This deficiency can be expected to have a serious effect on the development of classification systems for case-mix procedures.

Obviously also, an individual's disease may change from moment to moment, which requires that there be accurate recording of the time when a disease stage determination is made.

Each of these criteria is necessary and none of them in isolation is sufficient for disease definition. Although these criteria are medically meaningful, existing systems for the classification of disease (e.g., the International Classification of Disease Code) often fail to differentiate medical problems from diseases, and differentiations among diseases according to stage generally are overlooked. Such weaknesses in the system are of considerable significance in examining case-mix procedures for prospective reimbursement.[2,3]

SPECIFICATIONS FOR A CASE-MIX SYSTEM

The classification criteria for disease outlined earlier have obvious implications in the development of an appropriate case-mix system. However, there are multiple factors that affect a patient's length of stay in a hospital, the kinds of treatments administered, and the patient's response to treatment. A proper case-mix classification system requires the appropriate utilization of a medically sound disease classification as its starting point, but this may not be sufficient for all of the purposes to which the case-mix classification will be put.

An important issue is the extent to which the case-mix classification system separates different groups and the extent to which it combines them. If patients were to be classified in terms of many variables, homogeneous groupings might be found, but these might be irrelevant to the purposes of the system. Patients' ages, heights, geographical origins, and occupations clearly would be irrelevant, at least when taken in isolation. It is necessary to consider the relevance of the variables to the patients' diseases and to their responses to the treatments given.

Among the variables to be considered (beyond the obvious variable of their diseases), are (1) age, (2) sex, (3) expectations of the patients and of others, and (4) social support available to the patients. There may be interactions among these variables. For example, expectations may be different, depending upon the patient's disease and age. Social support available may in turn affect expectations. If medical treatment does not take into account these and other factors, significant problems may arise.

A crucial issue involves whether or not treatment for a given condition should be included among other variables for purposes of initial classification. Treatment should be thought of as an independent variable that may be studied in relation to the dependent variables, including patient condition and disease. Case-mix classi-fication should permit empirical studies to be made of different populations of patients with different diseases who have received different kinds of treatment (and for which different charges and medical costs are involved) in order to determine the treatments that are most cost-effective, taking into account multiple patient and social variables.

It is extremely important, of course, to examine both long-term and short-term results in such studies.[4] Hornbrook describes some of the criteria to be taken into account in selecting a case-mix system for reimbursement purposes.[5,6] Other factors that should be considered:

- Incidental health problems may affect how a patient responds to treatment for a given disease. A patient who has multiple health problems is different from one who has only one.

- The moment there is medical intervention, the nature of the health problem changes. Determination of an individual's health problem thus is a function of when an intervention occurs relative to the patient's disease.

- The quality of medical care given is important. If medical care has not led to desired results, this should be recognized and the reason(s) for the ineffectiveness should be studied.

- The incidence of disease in communities, or the frequency with which patients with certain health problems are seen at particular institutions, should be recognized as affecting the availability of health care resources and how they are used.

In addition, what may be called negative criteria that nevertheless are used for case-mix classification for health care reimbursement purposes should be recognized:

- Classification should not be made on the basis of resources actually expended in providing care but on resources that should have been used.

- Consideration should not be limited to what services have been provided for a patient at a given time without also determining whether or not additional services were required in the treatment in the near or even distant future for the same or a related condition.

- Readmission of the patient to the same or to another institution for the same health problem should lead to questions as to the effectiveness and efficiency of the original treatment.

Ultimately, of course, the goal is a case-mix classification system that ensures effective treatment at minimal monetary (and other) costs. This should call for an experimental approach to the development of case-mix systems. Unfortunately, this has not been done. The fundamental proposition governing case-mix classification systems should be to ensure that patients with similar medical diseases under comparable other relevant circumstances should receive similar treatments, that they should have similar outcomes, and that reimbursements accordingly should be similar. The question is whether any measure of similarity is meaningful across different patients within a given disease category. It is the authors' opinion that within disease categories, properly phrased, meaningful comparisons may be made.

DRGs: DEFINITION, DESCRIPTION, CRITICISMS

The diagnosis related groups (DRGs) case-mix classification system is a set of 470 different categories based upon principal diagnoses, surgical procedures used in treatment, and other factors.[7] The system contains 23 general categories, categories 1-13 and 16 being oriented to organ systems, while categories 14, 15, and 17-22 reflect disease etiology. The 23rd is a miscellaneous category for cases that do not fit into the 22 others. The categories are not organized to reflect specific disease etiologies or the severity (stage) of the disease (often referred to as intensity). A method for considering the severity of disease will be developed. There has been growing recognition of the importance of considering severity of illness as a parameter with regard to the DRG system but no resolution of this problem has been accomplished by 1986.

While the classification system ostensibly is based on disease grouping, the categorization is affected by whether surgery (major or minor) is involved in a patient's care. Consideration in the classification is given to "complications" and to "comorbidities," but no attempt has been made to classify or rank these factors. Age (general categories being 0 to 17, 18 to 69, and over 70) is another variable. For instance, if a patient is 70 or older, that factor is considered a complication that moves the case into another classification category for reimbursement purposes.

The DRGs are not intended to be clinical descriptors but rather to be clinically coherent and to reflect patterns of resource utilization associated with different patient conditions, broad disease categories, and forms of treatment administered. As a case-mix classification system, the DRGs permit patients to be categorized for purposes of reimbursement under the assumption that those within a given category should require comparable amounts of health care resources to be utilized in their treatment.

If all patients are homogeneous within a grouping, it is reasonable to assume that the same amount of resources will be expended in treating each of them. Experience indicates, however, that this is not the case.[8] The DRG system recognizes this by asserting that each category is homogeneous but that the distribution of treatment charges incurred will take the form of a normal or bell-shaped curve. If the category were homogeneous in terms of the health problems of patients included within the category, the variation would reflect random error or unusual efficiency or inefficiency in providing care. Unusual efficiency would be rewarded by reimbursement in excess of expenditure and unusual inefficiency would be penalized by reimbursement less than actual expenditure.

Recognizing that there might be factors other than chance and simple inefficiency involved, outliers (i.e., individuals whose care involved significantly greater or lesser resource utilization than the majority of patients in a given institution within the same grouping) then could be identified and analyzed. While it would appear at first glance that care given to those individuals who required the use of more resources in their treatment had been performed less efficiently, the developers of the system did not speculate about the outliers, i.e., those individuals for whom the charges were less than the mean within the group. They seem thus not to have recognized that costs may be kept low for a variety of reasons other than efficiency or may be high for reasons other than inefficiency.

Lower costs may be associated with such factors as patient death early in the treatment process, inadequate treatment, and premature discharge. Higher costs may be associated with different diseases (and different stages of diseases) that all fall within the same homogeneous classification category. Administrators and others concerned with maximizing the hospitals' bottom line inevitably will find (and, no doubt, already have found) ways to improve their financial positions by capitalizing upon the naïvete implicit in the DRG system. In fact, a term has been created to describe this: DRG creep. Given a patient who might reasonably be classified in a particular DRG, efforts may be made to place the patient in another DRG for which reimbursement may be greater. Computer programs have even been written that will train the user to select financially more rewarding categories for different patients.

The following are criticisms that thus may be raised about the DRG system of prospective reimbursement.

Homogeneity

From a medical point of view, the DRGs fail to ensure homogeneity with regard to the disease entities being classified:

- They fail to accommodate the essential dimensions of disease definition, including specification of disease etiology, organ system(s) involved, and the severity of the patient's condition. Multiple ambiguities are allowed to arise. For example, should a patient with an infectious disease of the respiratory system be classified under DRG category #4, the respiratory system, or under DRG category #18, which covers infections?

- They assign an arbitrary classification to someone 70 or older as equivalent to having a complication or comorbidity, which is very questionable. Moreover, an individual may be both over 70 and also have a complication or comorbidity. This is not recognized as worthy of attention.

- They fail to recognize that the patient's status may (and almost certainly will) change continuously during hospitalization. If a patient is admitted with a relatively benign disease stage but is treated inappropriately and the disease progresses so that surgical intervention becomes indicated, the individual may be placed in another DRG that provides the institution with greater reimbursement than had the patient been effectively treated at the outset.

- They provide no assurance that admitting diagnoses will not be used in lieu of discharge diagnoses, especially if this will place patients in more remunerative reimbursement categories.

- They make no provision for determining whether a complication was or was not present upon admission and there is no means for distinguishing between a disease-related comorbidity and one that is not.

- They offer no coherent method for recognizing, classifying, or ranking disease complications—the greatest weakness of DRGs. The system is virtually oblivious to disease stage. There is no way of knowing whether patients treated with a given "disease" in one hospital are comparable in terms of that "disease" with patients in another hospital, nor that all patients treated within a given hospital for a given "disease" in fact have the same disease.

Medical vs. Surgical

Another serious weakness in the DRG system lies in its failure to separate medical and surgical treatments from the conditions for which the treatments are being given.

- The reason for partitioning cases into those treated medically and those treated surgically is not clear, except that the latter are likely to have greater lengths of stay and to incur greater charges for care. This system thus encourages surgical over medical treatment for what may be the same condition. That is to say that in terms of the medical problems presented by patients in two different DRGs, there may be actual homogeneity. Heterogeneity is introduced on an arbitrary basis—that of treatment.

- DRGs, insofar as they are based on actual utilization data, are likely to perpetuate what they are intended to reduce or to control. A fatal flaw in science is to mix data with conclusions. This, in fact, is what the DRGs do. Initially this flaw might not make a great amount of difference, but over time serious systemic effects could be expected to result from it. Because surgery accounts for most of the expenses in hospitals, the use of DRGs will assure that this state of affairs will continue indefinitely and even that the tendency will become more pronounced.

Although the DRGs allow variations in charges to be identified, they provide no information as to the reasons for such variations. If all of the patients within a category are medically homogeneous, the variation should be analyzed for reasons other than disease. However, there is good reason to question whether patients within a category are, in fact, homogeneous, and whether those in different categories are really medically different.

The essence of scientific research involves determining the nature of variation and examining its causes. If variation is found within a specific DRG, care should be taken not to assign a reason for this (i.e., inefficiency or ineffectiveness of care), or to take action on it before determining its scope, nature, and causes. (That is to say, the model just presented with regard to the essential characteristics of a disease can be applied in other areas beyond those of disease.) Among the causes of variation within a DRG, the following should be considered:

- Categorical differences may exist among the various disease entities being treated. In particular, there may be differences in the level of seriousness of the conditions even though they may share the same name.
- Differences may arise out of various patient factors, including the individuals' ability and willingness to accept treatment. There may be differences in the availability of social and medical support facilities for different groups of patients.
- Secondary health problems may affect the kinds of treatment offered and the responses to such treatments. For example, patients being treated for diabetes mellitus also may have asthma or cardiac problems that affect treatment.
- Differences may be found in the appropriateness of diagnoses that have been made. There may have been misdiagnoses of certain conditions that in turn will skew all of the remaining data.
- Differences may be found in the quality of care.

When reimbursement rates for different institutions within a given geographical region or across geographical regions are compared, still other factors come into play:

- variations in the level of training and competence of the physicians providing care
- the remoteness of hospital facilities, climatic factors, or variations in regional patterns of care and in patient population characteristics

- variable technological resources among institutions; some specialize in treating certain kinds of illness, others provide a full range of services.

Empirical studies clearly are needed to explain identified variations. One approach to such studies might depend upon grouping DRGs, themselves, into certain categories:

1. Surgical procedures could be grouped according to regions of the body involved in the surgery—for example, craniotomies or major chest procedures.
2. Surgical procedures could be grouped according to the specific organ involved, such as appendectomies and cholecystectomies.
3. Medical problems could be grouped according to treatment provided, such as septicemia and congestive heart failure.
4. Medical diagnoses could be grouped, including such categories as diabetes mellitus.
5. Nonspecific symptoms and signs could be grouped—for example, such maladies as red blood cell disorders.

Greater homogeneity could be expected in category 2 in that list than in category 1, and in category 4 than in category 3. Category 5 could mean almost anything. By recognizing such variations, misleading comparisons could be identified and avoided. The temptation to classify the least sick individual within a DRG that includes much sicker patients could be reduced. So, too, could the temptation to upgrade an illness by performing a surgical procedure.

STAGING: DISEASE MATRIX CASE MIX

An alternative to the DRG case-mix classification system is what may be called the disease matrix case-mix classification system (DMC). Software for disease staging has been commercially available for some time. Presently, at Jefferson Medical College, a retrospective study of patients admitted at different disease stages is underway with funding provided by the Kellogg Foundation. The main focus of the study is to determine correlates and causes of late-stage admission to the hospital. Attention also has been directed to making comparisons of categorizations utilizing the DRG and the DMC approach. Also, all multiple choice questions utilized on certifying examinations administered by the American Board of Family Medicine are being classified according to the DMC in order to ensure that a broad range of diseases and health care problems is covered by each examination and that the focus of the questions is not limited to late-stage illness. To attempt to undertake a similar categorization utilizing the DRGs would, of course, produce only confusion. The DMC depends upon the definition of disease outlined above in which there are four identified dimensions necessary for a disease to be specified: specific pathophysiological disease manifestations, specific organs or organ systems affected, specific etiological agents, and disease stage defined according to a particular model of disease progression. This has been widely referred to as the disease stage system of case-mix classification, although, of course, disease stage is only one component of the system.[9,10]

Because the DMC is defined in medically relevant terms, many problems associated with the DRG approach are avoided. The DMC also has multiple applications and implications beyond case-mix classification. A limitation of the DMC is that it increases homogeneity within defined disease categories but not necessarily across disease categories.

As in the DRG system, there are approximately 400 DMC disease entities. Because there are several stages of disease in the DMC system, users must work not with the 470 categories of the DRGs but with well over 1,000 disease categories. Such reclassifications would, of course, be based upon similarities across disease conditions, not upon treatment considerations, which could still vary greatly. Insofar as the DRG system eventually will have to accommodate disease severity in some fashion, this difference may not be as great as it would seem initially. Of course, also, the actual number of categories used in a limited period may be much smaller because some of the disease entities classified are relatively infrequent. Further, many of the disease conditions are rarely (appropriately) treated on an inpatient basis in their early stages, and since the final stage for most diseases is death, the effective number of disease categories needed to classify hospital patient populations is quite limited.

It also is possible that for reimbursement purposes, certain disease conditions as classified by the DMC can be collapsed. Nevertheless, there may be problems in hospitals where relatively small numbers of patients are treated. If it is found to be necessary to collapse different disease conditions, this can be done on a rational basis by combining different disease entities that affect the same body or organ system or are associated with a common etiological agent. Certain illnesses may have common characteristics in late stages, at least as far as reimbursement is concerned. This would reflect what may be called a convergent quality, which can be expected in the presence of certain systemic complications that may have common treatment implications in various disease conditions.

Thus, for example, under some conditions, septicemia that results from bacterial meningitis may be medically similar to septicemia from a decubitus ulcer or bacterial pneumonia. The DRG approach provides no means of differentiating between one septicemia and another, and septicemia is listed as a specific DRG. On the other hand, it is known medically that septicemia associated with decubitus ulcers has therapeutic implications different from septicemia resulting from a ruptured appendix.

In any event, the authors believe that the DMC approach allows more reasonable and greater homogeneity within diagnostic categories than has been achieved through the DRGs or alternative systems of case-mix classification. It also allows for meaningful comparisons to be drawn across diseases when appropriate and makes it possible to recognize situations where this should not be done.

The DMC may be represented by a three-dimensional graph so that any given disease can be located within one cell of the graph (Figure 4–1). One axis of the graph represents body organ systems, a second axis categories of etiological agents associated with given diseases, and a third axis disease stage (severity). Special attention should be directed to this third axis because disease stage has been overlooked rather systematically in other case-mix classification systems.

The disease-staging technique employs the same methodology as that used in oncology. Oncologists recognize that there are discrete stages in the course of neoplastic diseases that can be defined and detected clinically. The model used in the classification of oncologic disease utilizes five stages, that used in the DMC involves only four. Oncologic usages require that a patient be staged only once during the course of the disease while the DMC system permits multiple classifications. The stages as used in the DMC system thus reflect the severity of the disease at any given time and have clinical significance in terms of prognosis and choice of therapy to be used in treating a particular patient.

Nearly all hospitalized patients can be classified unambiguously through the DMC system. The four stages mentioned above can be generally described as follows:

Stage I: Conditions with no complications, or problems of minimal severity.
Stage II: Problems limited to an organ or organ system; significantly increased risk of complications.
Stage III: Multiple site involvement; generalized systemic involvement; poor prognosis.
Stage IV: Death.

Each specific disease is staged using this framework on the basis of objective clinical findings and standard diagnostic nomenclature. These medical staging criteria are then translated into coded criteria by assigning (coded) diagnostic labels appropriate to each stage. The coded criteria represent an objective quantitative method of measuring disease severity in terms of data already contained on the hospital discharge abstract, which generally is available in electronic form. Moreover, the ability to classify severity by stage does not depend upon actual utilization patterns.

Diseases were selected for classification with two objectives in mind: (1) to include the major diseases in each etiology body system class and (2) to cover the majority of admissions to typical short-term general hospitals in the United States.

Figure 4–1 Disease Matrix Case-Mix Classification

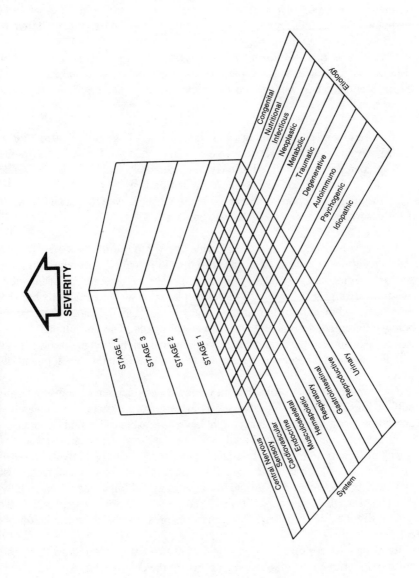
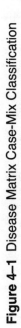

The first objective relates to the clinical meaningfulness and utility of the staging classification, while the second has implications in terms of administrative policy and for research purposes in health care settings.[11] The first step was achieved by calling upon a group of medical consultants with expertise in different areas of medicine. The second step involved analyzing diagnostic frequencies drawn from a sample of 387,000 discharge abstracts.

Twenty-three medical consultants participated in the specification of the staging criteria. Each disease was assigned to two consultants, who staged the disease independently. They were asked to define and to document their work in two categories:

1. A summary page defining each stage and substage was created. For each stage and substage a set of descriptors and synonyms for each descriptor was prepared. This provided criteria for objectively validating the presence of the disease and disease stage in a given patient.
2. References supporting the classification criteria were listed and a narrative description of the condition was prepared.

The consultants were required to divide every condition into at least four basic stage categories and were encouraged to develop as many substages within each primary staging category as they deemed appropriate on the basis of the medical literature. Each substage should place the patient at a significantly higher risk of morbidity and/or mortality than the previous substage and should be capable of being differentiated clinically from other substages. The consultants also were asked to specify etiology in all cases. The medical orientation in this classification activity is evident and can be contrasted with that used in the development of the DRGs.

The consultants were told that they should consider separate disease entities only, without regard for complications arising from possible simultaneous but unrelated conditions that patients might have (e.g., skin infection in a patient with hypertension), or their age. Finally, the consultants were instructed to define stages of disease in terms of biological complications only—infection, perforation, obstruction, hemorrhage, paralysis, shock, etc. Nonbiological factors, such as the patient's level of social functioning, emotional impairment, reaction to the disease, or occupational disability, were not to be considered except in the case of mental disease, where behavior was used to provide objective validation of the condition.

Each pair of consultants was assigned 20 to 30 conditions to stage. Each consultant returned the draft staging criteria to the chairperson, who reviewed the criteria for consistency with the staging guidelines. Any problems identified at this point were drawn to the attention of the consultant(s) and any differences between the two sets of criteria for each disease entity were discussed with each consultant working on the disease. The goal was to reach a consensus among the three individuals on the specification of the primary stages and substages. In some cases, other consultants with expertise in the particular disease area were called upon for opinions. Through this process, each criteria set was developed and reviewed by at least three physicians, two on an independent basis at first, then in a joint consensus process, with the physician panel chairperson participating in the development of all criteria to assure consistency.

Examples of sets of medical staging criteria for diabetes mellitus and for cholecystitis are presented in Tables 4–1 and 4–2.

CODED STAGING CRITERIA

To apply the medical staging criteria to large discharge abstract data bases, the medical criteria sets were translated into coded criteria. These were developed for use with the three most significant and widely used international diagnostic classification systems: ICDA-8, H-ICDA-2, and ICD-9-CM. Each statement in the medical criteria sets is represented by any or all possible codes or combinations of codes that reflect the conditions in that statement.

To accomplish the task of coding all the medical criteria into the three ICDA classification systems, consultants in the area of medical records review and with experience in the use of different coding systems were recruited from around the country. These medical records experts were given an explanation of the staging logic and instructions to be as inclusive as possible. Each criteria set was coded independently by two consultants, then reviewed by a third. This method provided a broad picture of coding styles and formats as well as the habits and behaviors of different coders.

Unfortunately, the ICD codes are not always sufficiently precise to capture the level of detail in the medical criteria. In a number of cases, one ICD code represents problems at more than one disease stage. In such cases, the code is assigned to the lower stage, thus understating the severity of the disease. This results in collapsing the higher stage into the lower stage. An example of this is found in the criteria for external hernia. Stage 2.1 is "irreducible hernia" and Stage 3.1 is "strangulated hernia." The ICD-9-CM codes for inguinal hernia with obstruction, without mention of gangrene (550.10–550.13), include inguinal hernia with incarceration, irreducibility, or strangulation. Therefore, this range of codes is included in the definition of Stage 2.1 because of the qualifying term "irreducible." Stage 3.1, strangulated hernia, then "collapses" to Stage 2.1 since the coding system does not specifically differentiate between irreducible and strangulated hernias.

Following the completion of the coding of the diseases by the two consultants, the two separate definitions were reviewed and a synthesis was developed. Sets of

Table 4–1 Sample Staging Criteria: Diabetes Mellitus

Stage	Common Description or Name of the Condition	Supporting Evidence or Clues
1.0	Diabetes mellitus	Normal history and physical, except for possibly history of polyuria–polydypsia; sugar elevation as defined. Fasting blood sugar greater than 110 MGM% or 2-hour postprandial greater than 140 MGM% and without ketoacidosis and without any other complications; or 2 random blood sugars greater than 140 MGM%
2.1	Diabetes mellitus with an infection in one or more systems (skin, genital tract, urinary tract infection, etc.)	Description and/or culture evidence of cutaneous skin infection: G.U. tract symptoms associated with infection—urgency, frequency, dysuria, cloudy, malodorous urine, hematuria, fever; lab results confirming infection: positive culture (cath or midstream), positive urine analysis, bacteria, WBC's, positive Gram stain. Infections include: pyoderma, impetigo, furunculosis, monilia of skin or vulva, cystitis, urethritis, epididymitis, prostatitis, pyelonephritis
2.2	Diabetes mellitus with acidosis, ketosis, ketonemia or ketonuria	Lab tests as defined plus elevated sugar and history: increased somnolence, fruity breath, fatigability and irritability, anorexia, diabetic ketoacidosis but without coma; serum pH less than 7.35 or CO_2 less than 23 mEq per liter and presence of acetone in serum
2.3	Diabetes mellitus with: Retinopathy but without loss of vision (microangiopathy) or Glomerulosclerosis without azotemia (Kimmelsteil-Wilson disease) or Neuropathy (peripheral or autonomic) or	—Fundoscopy: dilatation of veins, microaneurysms (usually, near macula), waxy exudates. At this stage no neovascularization or proliferative retinopathy —Usually asymptomatic albuminuria: assoc. elevation of BP may be due to renal lesion Peripheral neuropathy: —Sensory: loss of vibratory sense, paresthesias, pain —Neuromuscular: weakness, paralysis,

Table 4–1 continued

	Gangrene (tissue breakdown): arterial insufficiency with associated tissue breakdown	absent tendon reflexes, diabetic amyotrophy (thighs) Autonomic neuropathy: —Eye: extraocular muscle palsies, pupillary changes; —GI: decrease gastric emptying, GB dysfunction, nocturnal diarrhea; —GU: impotence, atony of bladder; —Vascular: orthostatic hypotension; —Skin: absent sweating, dependent edema, neurogenic ulcer History: claudication, trauma, evidence of neuropathy (painless foot); PE: pulseless foot. Characteristic changes in temperature and color
3.1	Diabetes mellitus with: Acidosis and coma (ketosis/ acidosis) or Retinopathy and loss of vision (proliferative retinopathy) or Necrotizing papillitis (papillary, medullary necrosis) or Azotemia or Septicemia	History: perhaps, no insulin in diagnosis Diabetic: nausea, vomiting, abdominal pain, labored breathing (Kussmaul), thirst. PE: dehydration, somnolence, relative hypotension, tachycardia Lab: as mentioned, plus inc. BUN, usually elevated potassium, inc. HCT., pH less than 7.3, CO_2 less than 10 mEq per liter. —As described in stage 2 plus neovascularization, proliferative retinopathy, and possibly retinal detachment —As described plus pyelonephritis, obstructive signs and symptoms; perhaps bacteremia, deteriorating renal function tests (papillae in urine or IVP evidence) —As stated plus acidosis (hyperphosphatemia, hypocalcemia), decreased serum pH and HCO_3, elevated serum K), anorexia, intermittent peripheral neuropathy, possible pericarditis, and uremic-hilar pneumonitis (BUN greater than 40 MGM% or creatinine greater than 3 MGM%)
3.2	Diabetes mellitus with hyperosmolar coma: non-ketotic, hyperosmolar hyperglycemic coma	History: decreased fluid intake, increasing somnolence, polyuria, average age 61; 40% new diabetes cases are noninsulin requiring. PE:

Table 4–1 continued

Stage	Common Description or Name of the Condition	Supporting Evidence or Clues
		rapid, shallow breathing, profound dehydration, obtunded to deep coma, often localizing neurological signs such as focal seizures. Lab: blood glucose average equals 1,096; only up to 2 plus serum acetone by acetest; HCO_3 (mEq/L) 17 plus or minus 5 (SD). Art. pH 7.26 (6.81-7.53), osmolarity 405 (348-456), BUN greater than 80mg/100 ml
3.3	Shock	
4.0	Death	

Reference:
Isselbacker et al. *Harrison's Principles of Internal Medicine* (New York: McGraw-Hill Book Company, 1980), p. 1741.

coded staging criteria for diabetes mellitus and cholecystitis are presented in Tables 4–3 and 4–4.

THE STAGING SOFTWARE

Once the coded staging criteria were complete, a software package was developed for assigning the stage of illness on the basis of diagnostic labels taken from standard hospital discharge abstract data. The software examines all diagnostic codes, sex, and discharge status.

The patient's record is staged for every disease category that is coded unless a given category can be combined with another (e.g., septicemia may be coded as a separate disease, but if the patient has a principal diagnosis of bacterial pneumonia or decubitus ulcer, septicemia would serve as a stage indicator for that principal diagnosis). The staging algorithms are designed to be so exhaustive collectively that a patient can always be assigned to at least one disease category. If the individual happens to have both appendicitis and diabetes mellitus, the presence and stages of both of these diseases will be identified by the staging software. The logic of this assignment is unambiguous since the coded staging criteria define precisely what conditions must be met for a patient to be classified with regard to any particular stage for any disease condition.

At the same time that these disease category and stage assignments are made, the software flags each of the staged diagnoses related to the patient's principal diagnosis by determining whether or not the principal diagnosis is associated with

Table 4–2 Sample Staging Criteria: Cholecystitis

Stage	Common Description or Name of the Condition	Supporting Evidence or Clues
1.0	Chronic cholecystitis: cholelithiasis	Abdominal x-ray, cholecystography, ultrasonography, computerized axial tomography, operation, pathological findings.
2.1	Chronic cholecystitis with choledocholithiasis (common duct stones)	Intravenous, transhepatic, intra-operative and endoscopic retrograde cholangiography, ultrasonography, computerized axial tomography, hepatic chemical profile, operation, pathological findings.
2.2	Acute cholecystitis	Abdominal x-ray, cholecystography, ultrasonography, operation, pathological findings.
2.3	Acute cholecystitis with choledocholithiasis (common duct stones)	Abdominal x-ray, cholangiography, hepatic chemical profile.
2.4	Gangrene of the gallbladder (necrosis of the gallbladder)	Operation, pathological findings.
2.5	Acute cholecystitis with localized perforation (pericholecystic abscess)	Abdominal x-ray, ultrasonography, operative findings, operative culture.
2.6	Empyema of gallbladder	Operation, pathological findings, culture of lumen and wall of gallbladder.
3.1	Gallstone ileus: cholecystoduodenal fistula; cholecystoenteric fistula	Abdominal x-ray, ultrasonography, operation, pathological findings.
3.2	Acute cholecystitis with acute suppurative cholangitis	Operation, pathological findings, culture of common bile duct.
3.3	Free (gross) perforation of gallbladder; bile peritonitis	Abdominal paracentesis, operation, pathological findings.
3.4	Acute cholecystitis and pancreatitis	Abdominal x-ray, ultrasonography, computerized axial tomography, blood and urine amylase.
3.5	Septicemia (specify organism) (biliary sepsis)	Blood culture.
3.6	Shock	Hypotension, tachycardia, oliguria, azotemia, acidosis.
4.0	Death	

Table 4–2 continued

NOTES

1. A. Wenckert and B. Robertson, "The Natural Course of Gallstone Disease," *Gastroenterology* 50 (1966): 376.
2. G.S. Kakos, R.K. Tompkins, W. Turnipseed, and R.M. Zollinger, "Operative Cholangiography," *Archives of Surgery* 104 (1972): 484.
3. M.H. Seltzer, E. Steiger, and F.E. Rosato, "Mortality Following Cholecystectomy," *S.G. Quarterly* 130 (1970): 64.
4. J.H.C. Ranson, "The Timing of Biliary Surgery in Acute Pancreatitis," *Annals of Surgery* 189 (1979): 654.
5. P. Malmstrom and A.M. Olsson, "Cholecystostomy for Acute Cholecystitis," *American Journal of Surgery* 126 (1973): 397.
6. L.W. Way and M.M. Sleisenger, "Cholelithiasis and Chronic Cholecystitis," in *Gastrointestinal Disease,* ed. M.M. Sleisenger and J.S. Fortran, vol. 2 (Philadelphia: W.B. Saunders Co., 1978), 1294–1302.
7. M. Korobkin and M.I. Goldberg, "Computerized Tomography of the Abdomen," in *Gastrointestinal Disease,* ed. M.M. Sleisenger and J.S. Fortran, vol. 2 (Philadelphia: W.B. Saunders Co., 1978): 1350–66.
8. G.R. Leopold, "Echography of the Abdomen," in *Gastrointestinal Disease,* ed. M.M. Sleisenger and J.S. Fortran, vol. 2 (Philadephia: W.B. Saunders Co., 1978): 1337–49.
9. L.W. Way and M.M. Sleisenger, "Choledocholithiasis, Cholangitis, and Biliary Obstruction," in *Gastrointestinal Disease,* ed. M.M. Sleisenger and J.S. Fortran, vol. 2 (Philadelphia: W.B. Saunders Co., 1978): 1313–25.
10. _____, "Acute Cholecystitis," in *Gastrointestinal Disease,* ed. M.M. Sleisenger and J.S. Fortran, vol. 2 (Philadelphia: W.B. Saunders Co., 1978): 1302–13.
11. J.A. MacDonald, "Perforation of the Gall Bladder Associated with Acute Cholecystitis," *Annals of Surgery* 164 (1966): 849.
12. J.D. McCarthy and J.C. Picazo, "Bile Peritonitis," *American Journal of Surgery* 116 (1968): 644.

---

any of the secondary diagnoses. This is a unique feature of the staging software made possible by the comprehensive definition of disease process embodied in the staging criteria.

In summary, based upon coded data, for each patient receiving treatment, as many separate diagnostic categorizations are made as may be indicated by the data. A primary staged condition is determined through review of the above information utilizing algorithms or rules generated in establishing the original disease staging criteria. Many of the secondary diagnostic categorizations thus become supporting evidence relative to the stage of the primary staged condition. The staging software has been written to operate on mainframe IBM computers and, depending on the hardware configuration, will process many hundreds of patient records per second. The software has been tested thoroughly and used to analyze several million discharge abstract records.

Table 4–3 Coded Sample Staging Criteria: Diabetes Mellitus

Stage	Common Description or Name of the Condition	ICD–9–CM Codes That Define Each Stage and Substage
1.0	Diabetes mellitus	775.10, 250.00–250.01, 250.80–250.91;
2.1	Diabetes mellitus with an infection in one or more systems (skin, genital tract, urinary tract infection, etc.)	S1.0 + 320.00–324.90, 245.00–245.10, 254.10, 289.20–289.30, 420.00–422.99, 424.91, 429.89, 447.60, 480.00–486.00, 510.00–510.90, 511.10, 513.00–513.10, 526.40, 566.00–567.90, 569.50, 572.00, 577.00, 580.81, 590.00–590.30, 595.00–595.40, 595.89–595.90, 597.00–597.80, 598.00–598.01, 599.00, 601.00–601.90, 603.10, 604.00–604.99, 607.10–607.20, 590.90, 608.00, 608.40–608.81, 611.00, 614.00–616.11, 616.30–617.90, 680.00–686.90, 711.00–711.99, 728.00, 730.00–730.39, 730.80–730.99;
2.2	Diabetes mellitus with acidosis, ketosis, ketonemia or ketonuria	S1.0 + 588.80, 791.60, 276.20–276.40; 250.10–250.11;
2.3	Diabetes mellitus with: Retinopathy but without loss of vision (microangiopathy) or Glomerulosclerosis without azotemia (Kimmelsteil-Wilson disease) or Neuropathy (peripheral or autonomic) or Gangrene (tissue breakdown); arterial insufficiency with associated tissue breakdown	S1.0–S2.2 + 337.10, 362.18, 443.81, 443.90, 446.60, 447.10, 581.81, 785.40, 354.00–356.90; 357.20, 362.01, 250.40–250.71;
3.1	Diabetes mellitus with: Acidosis and coma (ketosis/ acidosis) or Retinopathy and loss of vision (proliferative retinopathy) or	S2.3 + 276.20, 369.00–369.90; S1.0–S2.3 + 038.00–038.90, 583.70, 780.00, 790.60, 584.50–586.00, 590.80–590.81; 362.02, 250.30–250.31;

Table 4–3 continued

	Necrotizing papillitis (papillary, medullary necrosis) or Azotemia or Septicemia	
3.2	Diabetes mellitus with hyperosmolar coma; non-ketotic, hyperosmolar hyperglycemic coma	250.20–250.21;
3.3	Shock	S1.0–S3.2 + ZSHOCK9;
4.0	Death	S2.2–S3.3 + DEATH;

In contrast to other case-type classification systems, a significant characteristic of the staging approach is its emphasis on the medical meaningfulness of the criteria used. While numerous analyses have demonstrated the strong relationship between staging and resource consumption, it is important to emphasize that no utilization data were used to develop the staging criteria. This measure thus has an underlying a priori structure in which only the clinically pertinent attributes of the patient are employed.

While the shortcomings of the coding systems and discharge abstract process are well known, the reality is that most current health services' research, reimbursement approaches, and other activities dependent on case-mix measures are performed using computerized discharge abstract data bases. The development of coded versions of the staging criteria, and the staging software described, makes staging an efficient tool for analyzing these data bases.

Disease staging does not attempt to capture all the variables that contribute to hospital costs or resource utilization. Patient-related variables such as age, family support, or overall health status; provider-related variables such as choice of treatment modality; institutional capabilities such as the availability of special care units and teaching services; and community characteristics all can have significant impact on the cost and quality of care. These very important variables should be considered along with stage of illness when analyzing these issues.

It would indeed be surprising to find resource utilization and other factors the same across different groups of patients and different hospitals, given known variation in the variables cited. This variation permits studies to be made with regard to differences in patient outcome while the essential element of the health problems may be held constant.

Table 4–4 Coded Sample Staging Criteria: Cholecystitis

Stage	Common Description or Name of the Condition	ICD–9–CM Codes That Define Each Stage and Substage
1.0	Chronic cholecystitis; cholelithiasis	575.10, 574.00–574.21, 574.50–574.51;
2.1	Chronic cholecystitis with choledocholithiasis (common duct stones)	574.40–574.41;
2.2	Acute cholecystitis	575.00;
2.3	Acute cholecystitis with choledocholithiasis (common duct stones)	S1.0–S2.1 + S2.2; 574.30–574.31;
2.4	Gangrene of the gallbladder (necrosis of the gallbladder)	
2.5	Acute cholecystitis with localized perforation (pericholecystic abscess)	S1.0–S2.3 + 575.40;
2.6	Empyema of gallbladder	
3.1	Gallstone ileus; cholecystoduodenal fistula; cholecystoenteric fistula	560.31, 575.50;
3.2	Acute cholecystitis with acute suppurative cholangitis	
3.3	Free (gross) perforation of gallbladder; bile peritonitis	S1.0–S3.1 + 567.00–567.90, 614.50;
3.4	Acute cholecystitis and pancreatitis	S1.0–S3.1 + 577.00–577.10;
3.5	Septicemia (specify organism) (biliary sepsis)	S1.0–S3.4 + 038.00–038.90;
3.6	Shock	S1.0–S3.4 + ZSHOCK9;
4.0	Death	S2.2–S3.6 + DEATH;

COMPARISONS OF DRG AND DMC CASE MIXES

The differences between the DRG and DMC case-mix classification systems can be contrasted in terms of the assumptions upon which each depends. The assumptions upon which the DRGs are based may be stated as follows:

1. A single classification is made on the basis of organ system, general etiological category, or procedure that has been performed.

2. Variations within categories reflect inefficiency or ineffectiveness in patient care, at least if the variation is associated with increased utilization of resources.
3. Disease severity generally can be described in terms of the presence or absence of complications or comorbidities, all of which are equivalent in their medical significance. Age is equivalent to the presence of a complication or comorbidity; age and complications or comorbidity are not additive. Whether or not a complication appears during hospitalization or was present upon hospitalization is irrelevant.
4. Procedures utilized in providing treatment are an appropriate dimension for defining diagnostic categories. Reimbursement depends upon what is done to a patient, and not necessarily on how sick the person is or how effective the treatment procedures are.

On the other hand, the DMC case-mix classification system is based on the following assumptions:

1. Diagnostic categories for prospective reimbursement purposes reflect several dimensions associated with a medically meaningful disease model including etiology, organ or organ system affected, and stage of disease. Multiple categories may be required to describe a single patient.
2. Outliers do not necessarily indicate deficiencies in care; low levels of resource utilization may be indicators of greater potential problems in terms of quality of care than higher levels. Age is not necessarily a significant factor in measuring patient status.
3. Staging of different diseases is done precisely and following defined criteria.
4. Procedures utilized in providing treatment are not an appropriate dimension for defining diagnostic categories and are not so used.

A meaningful way of examining the strengths of these two case-mix systems is by comparing how they classify actual data. Such data are available and some examples are presented from a single study. Any institution can conduct similar studies electronically, using the staging software. Data presented here are for patients whose conditions were classified initially according to the DRG system and then were classified according to disease stage within DRG categories. This was done for all 470 DRG categories. Examples of what was revealed through this cross-classification activity are shown in Tables 4–5, 4–6, and 4–7. (It should be emphasized that in the absence of cross-classification as done here, it would be justifiable to assume that the patients included in each DRG category were homogeneous.)

The first DRG illustrates the major problem that has been attributed to the system—nonmedical homogeneity. Homogeneity exists only with regard to the

Table 4–5 Case-Mix Analysis: Severity within Diagnosis Related Groups
Stratified by Disease and Severity

DRG = 1: Craniotomy Age > = 18 Except for Trauma

Diagnosis	Stage	Count	Pct.	ALOS	Avg. Chg.
Cerebral Tumors	1	12	17.6	27.7	$10,408
Cerebral Tumors	4	2	2.9	14.5	7,155
Infratentorial Tumor of Brain	1	9	13.2	28.6	11,801
Defects of CNS (Brain &					
Spinal Cord)	3	8	11.8	18.8	5,448
Other Nervous System Conditions	1	3	4.4	9.7	4,094
Disease of Basilar Artery	2	1	1.5	54.0	17,290
Aneurysm of Cerebral Vessels	2	11	16.2	18.1	8,713
Aneurysm of Cerebral Vessels	3	8	11.8	42.9	20,779
Aneurysm of Cerebral Vessels	4	5	7.4	35.0	19,236
Disease of Vertebral Artery	2	1	1.5	18.0	6,931
Disease of Vertebral Artery	4	1	1.5	3.0	5,122
Essential Hypertension	3	4	5.9	32.0	11,805
Other Cardiovascular Conditions	1	2	2.9	115.0	42,165
Cancer of the Breast	4	1	1.5	13.0	7,026
Total DRG		68	100.0	28.8	12,168

fact that a common procedure was performed with regard to all of the patients involved (craniotomy), although this also may be argued. Patients included in this category were 18 or over and trauma is excluded as a reason for the procedure being performed. With regard to the categories mentioned earlier, craniotomy is a surgical procedure performed on a region of the body; considerable variation thus would be expected within this category in terms of length of stay and charges incurred, although the category was created in order to maximize homogeneity and, on the basis of such homogeneity, a constant reimbursement for all patients is provided.

Sixty-eight patients were included in this category. Their average length of hospital stay was 28.8 days and the average charge was $12,168. If a particular patient's care involved greater charges, the hospital lost the difference and, conversely, if the care involved lesser charges, the hospital pocketed the difference. Indeed, totals ranged from a low of $4,094 to a high of $42,165. The data presented refer to admissions during fiscal year 1980-1981 and are therefore considerably lower than would be expected with current charges.

On the face of it, using the reasoning implicit in the DRG system, there obviously is something wrong here. It would appear that one physician was ten times more efficient than another (although conceivably it is the same physician

Table 4–6 Case-Mix Analysis: Severity within Diagnosis Related Groups Stratified by Disease and Severity

DRG = 55: Miscellaneous Ear, Nose & Throat Procedures

Diagnosis	Stage	Count	Pct.	ALOS	Avg. Chg.
Serous Otitis Media	1	2	1.0	1.5	$ 952
Otitis Media	1	9	4.6	2.2	1,349
Otitis Media	2	5	2.6	1.8	1,093
Cholesteatoma	1	3	1.5	2.0	1,543
Purulent Sinusitis, Nasal Sinuses	1	1	0.5	1.0	812
Anaerobic Infections	1	1	0.5	2.0	1,014
Laryngeal Papillomas	1	8	4.1	3.3	1,439
Cancer of Glottis	1	3	1.5	3.0	1,045
Hearing Loss due to Otosclerosis	1	18	9.2	2.4	1,303
Meniere's Disease	1	1	0.5	4.0	2,068
Hypertrophy of Tonsils and Adenoids	1	2	1.0	1.5	751
Other EENT Conditions	1	125	63.8	2.6	1,497
Croup—Viral & Epiglottitis	1	2	1.0	6.5	4,077
Parainfluenza Viral Disease	1	2	1.0	4.0	2,945
Coxsackie and ECHO Virus Infections	1	1	0.5	2.0	955
Cancer of Hypopharynx	1	1	0.5	3.0	1,138
Disease of Salivary Glands	2	1	0.5	3.0	1,508
Fracture of: Maxilla	1	10	5.1	1.9	997
Other Musculoskeletal Conditions	1	1	0.5	1.0	983
Total DRG		196	100.0	2.6	1,446

with two different patients). Similarly, the average length of stay varied between three days for one group of patients and 115 days for another. If the average length of stay is 28.8 days, one physician is nine times more efficient than the average and another is four times less efficient.

However, examination of patient data utilizing the DMC and staging approaches indicates that several different conditions were being treated with craniotomy and, for each of these, patients were being treated in different disease stages. One of the craniotomy patients was identified as having a diagnosis of cancer of the breast. The charges for this patient were $7,026, so the hospital "made" more than $5,000 in comparison with the average craniotomy charge of $12,168. (Had the patient been included in the category of malignant breast disorders (DRG #274), the average charge would have been $5,333 and the hospital would have lost nearly $2,000.)

Table 4–7 Case-Mix Analysis: Severity within Diagnosis Related Groups
Stratified by Disease and Severity

DRG = 69: Otitis Media & URI Age 18–69 W/O C.C.

Diagnosis	Stage	Count	Pct.	ALOS	Avg. Chg.
Dementia	3	1	4.0	8.0	$1,832
Serous Otitis Media	1	1	4.0	4.0	1,048
Otitis Media	2	2	8.0	5.5	1,099
Streptococcal Pharyngitis	1	3	12.0	3.0	1,346
Streptococcal Pharyngitis	2	3	12.0	3.3	866
Purulent Sinusitis, Nasal Sinuses	1	3	12.0	3.0	931
Anaerobic Infections	1	1	4.0	2.0	882
Other EENT Conditions	1	4	16.0	3.8	1,640
Parainfluenza Viral Disease	1	3	12.0	3.3	1,114
Influenza	1	2	8.0	2.0	1,075
Coxsackie and ECHO Virus Infections	1	1	4.0	3.0	756
Chronic Lymphocytic Leukemia	2	1	4.0	3.0	1,115
Total DRG		25	100.0	3.5	1,172

Other conditions included in DRG 1 were: (1) cerebral tumors, (2) defects of the central nervous system, (3) aneurysm of cerebral vessels, and (4) essential hypertension. In general, stage 2 or 3 conditions within a given disease category cost substantially more than stage 1 or 4 conditions. It might be inferred that, from a strictly financial point of view, hospitals would do well to take patients who were not seriously ill (i.e., stage 1) or who died while in the hospital (stage 4) provided, of course, that death was relatively rapid.

Similarly, DRG 55 identifies a wide assortment of specific diseases within the category of miscellaneous ear, nose, and throat procedures (see Table 4–6). Although nearly all of the patients in the sample are in stage 1 of their respective illnesses, the average charge to the hospital per patient varied between $751 and $4,077, with the average for all groups being $1,445. On the other hand, in DRG 69 (otitis media and upper respiratory infection for patients between 18 and 69 without complications) who had multiple diagnoses and several stages, the variation is slight—ranging from $756 to $1,640.

These DRG data, if examined uncritically, would indicate that certain physicians were inefficient or that their treatments were ineffective. What appears to be happening is that understandable variations arising from heterogeneity in the classification system are being ignored. If these data are typical, and there is reason to believe they are, the DRG system clearly fails the test of medical homogeneity and can result only in serious distortions in the reimbursement system for services and ultimately in the health care system as a whole.

Unfortunately, institutions may find it useful to classify patients so that hospital income is maximized. It is possible in the DRG system for a hospital to alter its case mix by stressing the diagnosis that calls for the highest rate of reimbursement or on the basis of which procedure was performed without regard to the patient's condition. If a hospital makes money when surgery is performed, surgical procedures may be used where the patient might be better treated medically. The hospital may decide to admit only the less sick patients in a given category of illness and pass the more seriously ill on to other institutions. The possible effects of this on the operation of hospitals and on the health care of society could be staggering. What is perhaps most distressing is that these problems are obvious and have been recognized over a considerable time while other options that would aid hospitals in avoiding these outcomes have been available but have not been used.

It is not unlikely that certain institutions will concentrate on certain diseases because of what are called economies of scale, and certain disease categories associated with small profit and inefficiency of operation will be virtually phased out. This may include emergency department services and certain kinds of care (e.g., burn units) that are used irregularly and unpredictably but that require high overhead. What will happen to these patients in communities that have no hospitals willing to provide these services?

OTHER APPLICATIONS OF DISEASE CASE MIX

In addition to its utility as a case-mix classification system, staging or DMC has a number of other uses:

- Quality of care assessment: The DMC can provide data related to the level of severity of illness that, in turn, can give an indication of problems in quality of care in ambulatory settings. It leads to the development of hypotheses regarding the cause(s) of undesirable health outcomes. Are they the result of patient, physician, institutional, or community-related problems?[8,10,11]

- Facility planning: The DMC can provide data concerning the level of severity of specific patient groups (e.g., those with cardiovascular disease) that may warrant the establishment or expansion of special care units or acquiring special diagnostic equipment or other facilities.

- Professional staffing in health care institutions: The data may indicate the appropriateness or inappropriateness of present or planned personnel levels in hospitals in relation to patients' actual needs.

- Medical education: Undergraduate, graduate, and continuing medical education may be based upon an application of staging concepts. For example, to what extent does the curriculum in the medical school address late stage illness and early stage illness? How much attention is devoted to problems associated with particular body organ systems or of a particular etiological nature?

- Clinical trials: Medical research may be conducted more meaningfully if subjects for studies are homogeneous in terms of their health problems. Staging permits better definition of such homogeneity. This may be especially important when reports of the usefulness of various medications for different conditions are reported or when there is concern about negative side effects of such medications.

- Professional credentialling: Physicians and other health professionals may develop expertise in limited areas of medicine. The DMC approach provides a better way of defining such expertise. This may be of great value in helping professionals recognize their limitations and deficiencies. A surgeon who is very competent in managing stage 2 patients may be quite inadequate for those with stage 3 illness, depending, perhaps, upon the particular ailment. Such individuals are by no means incompetent. However, the DRG system may contribute to incompetence and inefficiency as some individuals may be encouraged to provide care to patients whose conditions may not even require hospital treatment.

FUTURE DIRECTIONS

One of the most difficult things for policymakers to do is to acknowledge errors in their initial ideas and assumptions. It may be inferred from this notion that in all likelihood it will be necessary to live with the DRG case-mix classification system for the foreseeable future in spite of its obvious deficiencies and limitations. Speculation is possible as to the reasons for the federal government's rapid and apparently uncritical acceptance of DRGs.

There is no doubt that the system is beneficial to certain groups of professionals and to certain institutions, and may seem to control costs if patient outcomes are not monitored carefully. However, by differentiating between surgical and non-surgical care, which the DRGs do, they tend to preserve the status quo. They are likely to do so, however, at the expense of individuals whose need for medical services may be the greatest—those in stages 2 and 3 of their diseases. The system definitely will affect the economic well-being of large teaching hospitals, which are more likely to have sicker patients. What will happen to the poor, who are more likely to be more seriously ill? Who will deal with the ethical and social issues that will emerge? How will medical education be affected?

It is to be hoped that some changes will be introduced into the DRG case-mix system to make it more meaningful medically. At the very least, staging concepts should be used to analyze outliers and to justify making exceptions for reimbursement purposes. In addition, the data provided by staging of diseases are essential elements for hospitals' management of their resources. This will produce a patchwork quilt effect that will function much less well than had a system of disease classification more meaningful medically been used from the outset.

Attention also needs to be directed to the measurement of medical care effectiveness. This may be accomplished by measuring and analyzing patient data at multiple points in the health care cycle. These include medical status upon admission to the hospital, status during the stay, and status at discharge. This approach will allow hospital managers and physicians to do cost analysis consistent with medical logic.

Finally, if physicians are to be paid under a case-mix reimbursement system on a predetermined or prospective basis, essential characteristics of disease (i.e., etiology, organ system affected, and stage) must be accommodated within the classification system.

Were these recommendations to be accepted, the results could provide data necessary to evaluate medical education and to influence public policy in the health care field on a broad basis, including reimbursement.

NOTES

1. Joseph S. Gonnella, "Patient Case Mix: Implications for Medical Education and Hospital Costs," *Journal of Medical Education* 56, No. 7 (July, 1981): 610–611.

2. Mark C. Hornbrook, "Hospital Case Mix: Its Definition, Measurement, and Use: Part I. The Conceptual Framework," *Medical Care Review* 39, No. 1 (Spring, 1982a): 1–43.

3. Mark C. Hornbrook, "Hospital Case Mix: Its Definition, Measurement and Use: Part 2. Review of Alternative Measures," *Medical Care Review* 39, No. 2 (Summer, 1982b): 73–123.

4. Joseph S. Gonnella, et al., "Use of Outcome Measures in Ambulatory Care Evaluation," in *Ambulatory Medical Care Quality Assurance,* ed. G.A. Biebink and H.H. White (La Jolla, Cal.: La Jolla Health Science Publications, 1977), pp. 91–125.

5. Hornbrook, 1982a.

6. Hornbrook, 1982b.

7. R.B. Fetter, et al., *The New ICD-9-CM Diagnosis Related Groups Classification Scheme: Users Manual,* Volume 1 (New Haven: Yale University, School of Organization and Management, Health Systems Management Groups, 1981).

8. Mohan L. Garg, et al., "Evaluating Inpatient Costs: The Staging Mechanism," *Medical Care* 16, No. 3 (March, 1978): 191–201.

9. Joseph S. Gonnella, Mark C. Hornbrook, and Daniel Z. Louis, "Staging of Disease: A Case-Mix Measurement," *Journal of the American Medical Association* 251, No. 5 (February 3, 1984): 637–644.

10. Joseph S. Gonnella, Daniel Z. Louis, and James J. McCord, "The Staging Concept: An Approach to the Assessment of Outcome of Ambulatory Care," *Medical Care* 14, No. 1 (January, 1976): 13–21.
11. Joseph S. Gonnella and Carter Zeleznik, "Factors Involved in Comprehensive Patient Care Evaluation," *Medical Care* 12, No. 11 (November, 1974): 928–934.

Chapter 5

The Adequate Patient Record

Carolyn Anderson-Stewart

adequate (ad'i-qwit) adj. 1. to be able to satisfy a requirement; suitable. (Lat. adaequatus, p. part. of adaequare, to equalize; ad-to + aequare to make equal.)

American Heritage Dictionary

When defining the phrase "adequate patient record," the question is: "Adequate for whom and for what purpose?" What data collection requirements must be met? How much documentation is needed to provide information that will meet those requirements? Does the word "adequate" have the same meaning for all users? What does the word adequate mean to the creators of the information? What does it mean to the users? Clear answers to these questions must be provided. The creators and users of the record must understand clearly who is going to use it and for what purpose.

Many health care providers and consumers are interested in what is contained in patient health records. Decision makers in finance, medicine, consumer and government groups, and health care professionals all request access to such information. Financial, clinical, administrative, and governmental decisions often are based on such information. Through the use of data abstracted from clinical records and used in research projects, decisions can be made that will affect the overall health and life style of citizens. Important conclusions with far-reaching economic and social impact may be based upon the patient's diagnosis, treatment, and outcome as shown in the patient's record.

Such agencies as the Food and Drug Administration (FDA) and the Centers for Disease Control (CDC) publish findings that influence formation of public policy. Many of these findings are based on data and information collected from patient records as well as directly from epidemiological studies. The implications for the use of the record by such a variety of policymaking groups demand that the documentation accurately describe health care episodes.

In a health facility, the management of institutional resources often is dependent upon the documentation in the record. A simple note recording the date and time of admission and of discharge may make the difference between a reimbursement that is equitable and one that does not cover the cost of services. Omission of a note reporting a complicating condition that may have justified an extended length of stay can make a difference in reimbursement.

In direct patient care, providers carefully document orders, treatment, and results in order to evaluate the effectiveness of treatment and the quality of care. Physicians carefully select the treatment modality they believe in their professional judgment to be the best for patients with given diagnoses. By documenting the protocol or treatment plan and its results, providers may be able to determine the effectiveness of that care. The appropriateness of the care may be studied by reviewing physician practice as documented in the record.

As patients move from provider to provider or from institution to institution, the information that describes their health status should accompany them. The importance of tracking such health services is obvious; continuity of care is best provided when prior information about condition and treatments, with outcomes, is available. Given the variety of persons who assist patients with medical, financial, social, and emotional problems, the record information must be comprehensive, accessible, and easily understood.

The adequate clinical document—the patient record—must be one containing the information needed by a variety of users to provide comprehensive care, to evaluate its delivery and appropriateness, and to make administrative decisions about it. Information needs of groups of users differ. What is adequate or suitable for one group may not be for the needs of another. But whatever the use of the record, there must be a clear understanding of who is to use it and for what purpose. There must be assurance that the users understand what is being recorded and that the language is clear and means the same thing to both the users and the creators. Therefore, it is critical that the selection of data elements or of information for the record be managed carefully, that a consensus be reached on what is to be included and how it is defined, and that its use is encouraged. It is one thing to provide the definition; it is another thing to have it used.

SELECTION OF DATA ELEMENTS

The selection of data elements or information used to describe the health status of individuals should be made by the professional groups that will be entering those data into the record. With participation in the selection of elements and agreement on meanings, the users and creators share a kind of commitment to the integrity of the patient information. In the design of any health care information system, identification of data needs for patient profiles must be made by users at outset. Questions to be addressed include: Why are these data needed? What is the purpose for collecting such data? What kind of health care reports will be generated from these data?

In answering such questions, care should be given to understanding the use of individual as well as aggregate data collected by federal and state agencies. Each element should contribute to the development of individual patient financial, social, and medical profiles as well as institutional and professional staff performance profiles. Data must be capable of movement from specific to aggregate.

Numerous basic data sets have been developed and validated. To these may be added data elements that are specific to a region and/or an institution. Use of the validated data sets accomplishes two things:

1. Valid comparisons among and between health care providers may be possible.
2. Individual providers who use the minimum data set will not have to develop their own and may concentrate instead on acquiring additional data to address their unique needs.

Regardless of the similarity of need or difference among the elements, the definitions must be understood, must be unambiguous, and must be commonly held.

In 1975 the National Committee on Vital and Health Statistics Related to Patient Care Data established a consultant panel to review recommendations for uniform minimum health data sets. "Uniform minimum health data set—An array of specified information elements and their standardized definitions developed for a specific purpose that are regularly collected by agreement among institutions and individuals providing health care services, regardless of the specific format or form on which they are reported."[1] National data sets have been established with the underlying strategy of limiting as much as possible the development of data elements needed by the majority of users.

These data sets were developed to provide baseline statistics for the following general functions or purposes:

- evaluation of the extent and expense of service
- management of health care institutions, agencies, and services
- public monitoring and regulation of services
- health planning and policymaking
- education of health personnel
- research to define health care problems.

The data sets have been weighted carefully in relation to the primary requirements of various groups of users. Each element has been justified in terms of its precise applications by a substantial number of user groups. However, the scope of national data sets and the multiple uses for which they are intended are only minimums. Groups of users developing new data sets and elements for patient records or inpatient discharge data may want to add to these minimums. Individuals working on sets of elements that are extensions of these minimum sets will recognize that many desirable data elements and subcategories have been omitted in an effort to limit the size of the generic set. Designers of new data systems should consider their specific needs before expanding any of the national data sets, bearing in mind not only the users and the purpose for collecting the information but also the substantial costs in staff time and money in collecting and processing data.

NATIONAL DATA SETS

The following summary reviews each nationally developed data set and its current status of implementation.[2]

Uniform Hospital Discharge Data Set (UHDDS)

The Uniform Hospital Discharge Data Set is the product of the 1969 conference on Hospital Discharge Abstract Systems.[3] The UHDDS defines elements that all short-term general hospitals should collect on all discharges. The UHDDS (1984) is being used in federal health programs as part of (1) Uniform Bill–82 (UB–82), (2) Medicaid Management, (3) Integrated Data Management Systems, (4) Professional Review Organization (PRO), (5) Prospective Payment, (6) National Hospital Discharge Survey, (7) Indian Health Board, (8) Veterans Administration, and (9) Department of Disease. Although the UHDDS is being used by these organizations, there are minor modifications in the inclusion or exclusion of certain elements. Some organizations have different definitions for the items.

Ambulatory Care Minimum Data Set (ACMDS)

The Ambulatory Care Minimum Data Set data elements were recommended as a result of the 1972 Conference on Ambulatory Care Data.[4] These are divided into two segments: (1) registration data to be collected for each patient initially and updated as needed, and (2) encounter data to be collected for each patient visit. This minimum data set is not known to be in use in any of the programs in the Department of Health and Human Services (DHHS) or in any other federal agency. However, with increased emphasis on ambulatory care in lieu of inpatient hospitalization, the use of the Ambulatory Care Minimum Data Set may occur.

Long-Term Care Minimum Data Set (LTCMDS)

This data set was developed at a 1975 conference cosponsored by Johns Hopkins University and the National Center for Health Studies (NCHS).[5] The conference participants outlined a data set consisting of 24 elements, of which 12 were included in substantially the same form in the hospital discharge and/or ambulatory care minimum data set. The importance of the data set has been recognized by users other than DHHS; the Veterans Administration uses it in the information system of its hospital-based Home Care Program.

Health Facilities Minimum Data Set (HFMDS)

The Health Facilities Minimum Data Set was designed originally in response to the need for data collection through the Cooperative Health Statistics System (CHSS) of the National Center for Health Studies.[6] The potential health facility users were listed as: CHSS-covered hospitals, nursing homes, and other care facilities (homes for the blind, deaf, emotionally disturbed, dependent children, unwed mothers, mentally retarded, physically handicapped, and resident treatment centers for alcoholics and drug abusers). As far as can be determined, this set is not being used by any organization or agency.

Health Professional Minimum Data Set (HPMDS)

The Health Professional Minimum Data Set was developed to establish a systematic national program for collecting comparable data on the supply of health professionals.[7] The extent to which states are continuing to collect minimum data set items for various health professionals is not known. While all of these minimum sets have been developed for intended use by the federal government to collect comparable data across geopolitical lines, many have been discarded or are used only in part, mostly because of budget constraints. However, to data set developers these may serve as a beginning for identifying elements that individual institutions and groups may wish to use in preparing their patient records.

Language As a Factor

Regardless of the minimum data set or additional data elements that may be needed by various user groups, creators and developers must make decisions about what to record and what to omit. The key to developing adequate patient records is not so much to assemble great amounts of documentation but rather to provide the applicable and appropriate documentation through the discriminating use of language to define each episode narrowly. Does the language or nonverbal symbol convey what it is meant to convey?

When considering adequate patient records, some thought must be given to the use of language as a means of communication. This may be a separate issue from data element identification and definition process but may contribute to the decision on the extent to which narrative records should be maintained. Narratives tend to be highly descriptive accounts of patient care; the best-known example is Nurses Notes. Narratives can provide information missing from a collection of data elements; therefore, it is generally thought that some narrative must be included in the record if it is to be complete and adequate. The questions are: What constitutes a narrative? How much narrative should be included? Where should it be located in the record? What do words in the narrative mean to users? Do the same words have the same meanings for all users?

Kritek reports that, for nursing alone, there are numerous language systems used to create narratives.[8] The most common of these, because of its long tradition of dominance in the practice of health care, is the language developed by the medical community, i.e., medical terminology.

Kritek adds that a second set of languages may emerge from various specialties within nursing. Some are linked directly to medical specialties, such as orthopedics. Various academic specialties in nursing such as education, anthropology, and physiology also prompt use of language appropriate to those disciplines. Nurses prepared in education speak of learning objectives; those in anthropology, of folk health beliefs; those in physiology, of electrolyte imbalance.[9] Kritek observes that the language most important to delivery of direct patient care is that used by practicing nurses. The integral components of nurses' language appear to be those of utility.

Other health care professionals similarly prepared may have developed their own sets of language. Physiatrists and physical therapists often describe patient care in behavioral terms similar to those used by nursing. Language must describe what is understood to be happening. The selection of language to describe medical or health care events requires that both sender and receiver have the same understanding. When the sender and the receiver are of the same profession, same culture, or same ethnic group, understanding is more likely to occur than when they are not.

This holds true not only for the information flow between professionals but also between consumers and providers. Physicians speak of patients who have difficulty understanding questions so that it is not possible to obtain useful answers. The history of illness or clear identification of complaint may be lacking. To obtain complete information, an interview process often must be followed. Interview techniques definitely influence data completeness and accuracy.[10] The creation of an adequate clinical document may be dependent upon the interviewer's asking the right questions, recognizing useful answers, and acting upon that information. The record is composed of language that is understood clearly, professional to professional and provider to consumer.

In sum, the adequate clinical record describes the total patient experience either in narrative elements or in signs and symbols; the language is succinct yet comprehensive, descriptive yet spare.

The decision as to when to utilize isolated data elements that may be organized and retrieved by computer, or when to turn to lengthy narrative in the record, requires professional judgment. A situation may be described best using numbers or symbols, at other times with the narrative description.

If the purpose of collecting the data has been determined before the selection of data elements and the design of the record, the developers will be guided by that purpose when choosing a format.

THE COMPUTERIZED RECORD

In the majority of health care institutions, the clinical document is a paper record. Through the use of multiple forms, checklists, outlines, and multiple-choice formats, paper reports are generated and arranged into the patient record. Inpatient records describe individuals' institutional stays; outpatient records describe visits as chronological reports of face-to-face encounters.

Over the years, the number of forms and amount of narrative content in the patient record has increased so that now it is not uncommon to have records of 60 or more pages per hospital stay and volumes of pages for continuing outpatient visits. Often, specific information needed for patient care, administrative decisions, or research is scattered throughout the pages of the record and is difficult to locate. As the need for information increases, in part because of the anticipated accountability for expanded practice, the accessibility, accuracy, and completeness of the information is of primary importance.

Manually prepared records and methods of documentation may no longer be effective, and computer-generated data in alternative formats may be the method chosen to provide timely and accurate descriptions.

With the advent of the computer and its application to health care, accessibility of information should be easier. The paper health record may be replaced gradually by the paperless or computerized health record. In many institutions, the transition has begun and information formerly documented on paper is being keyed into computers. The patient record may be viewed on the cathode ray tube (CRT) screens and paper copies made of selected reports. This new record is designed to provide data needed for patient management, administrative decisions, and research in succinct, logically sequenced formats that are readily accessible to users. If narrative descriptions are preferred, limited space may be provided on the CRT screen.

The technology of the computer permits the creation and use of individually tailored record arrangements for thousands of patients. Through the computers' extensive storage capacity, individual records may include more patient/treatment specific data than ever before. The records may truly describe the uniqueness of each patient. Generalizations are possible using aggregate data and patient-specific issues are addressed through use of individual data. It may be possible to answer questions such as: ''Why does Patient A respond differently to a treatment than Patient B, given that most variables in individuality affecting outcome are the same?'' Or, ''Is it possible that ethnicity may have a role in determining how patients respond to treatment?'' Treatment selection tailored specifically to individual needs may be possible.

It is important to recognize that although an average response to treatment may be observed, professionals must be prepared for the exception; patient-specific data will provide information for dealing with such exceptions. The patient record—the adequate clinical document—must have the capacity to delineate ways in which people are exceptional or how they differ (e.g., in response to treatment). Data unique for individuals may be recorded in the computer.

Recording information electronically and in standardized formats provides data elements and language that are clearly defined, understood, and utilized properly, minimizing chances for error. The problems of poor handwriting, inappropriate use of language, and excessive volume of narrative information are minimized with the computerized record. For example, computer printouts of laboratory test results reduce the amount of paper by eliminating single sheets that may cover only one or two test results. With the totally computerized record, laboratory reports may be found on the screen and a paper report of selected reports generated as needed. Computer printouts offer more concise and readable data for record users.

Some caution should be exercised when using computerized records. They are only as useful and adequate as the data they contain. Ideally, the creators of the elements—that is, those who define practice—should be the persons who understand the actions and the meaning of the language, signs, and symbols that describe those actions. To minimize the chance for error, data should be entered at the closest point of action, preferably by the person completing the action.

Every precaution should be taken to allow for variability in practice, that is, the standardized format should not dictate standardized treatment, but should allow for individual patient responses and reactions to treatments. When the data collection process and the patient record become standardized for computer compatability, both patient individuality and opportunities for variability in medical practice may be lost; the data collection method and elements could dictate the protocol for patient care, possibly ignoring the uniqueness of individual response to treatment. The standardized computer compatible format should not dictate standardized treatment.

The greatest benefit in using the computerized record may be the opportunity to provide current, day-to-day data that are entered and utilized almost simultaneously. When the patient is discharged, the final record will be available to assure continuity of care without having to be assembled, analyzed, and reviewed for completion, although those activities should occur some time during the data entry process.

THE ADEQUATE RECORD AS FINANCIAL TOOL

In this age of cost efficiency and fiscal accountability, the patient record, along with various cost accounting, order entry, and financial reports, has taken on new importance. The language of health care formerly reserved for use in delivering services has now become the language that supports the payment received for those services. This language may be as unknown to financial experts as any foreign tongue. Yet financial personnel are making economic decisions on payment for health care services based on information that has been recorded in the patient record as the language of medicine or nursing or some other health care specialty.

The new challenge for health care practitioners and providers lies in extending the understanding of the health care language to the outside world, to users beyond the walls of the health care institution. It is crucial to the economic well-being of the social system that knowledge and understanding of the language on which financially significant health care decisions are made extend to other users.

STANDARDS FOR DOCUMENTATION

Various state and private licensing and accrediting bodies require that certain standards for documentation be met in order to have the hospital accredited. The adequate clinical record must meet these standards while continuing to provide data needed for patient care, administrative decisions, and research. These standards usually are provided in the form of manuals and state administrative codes.

Although codes may vary from state to state, the federal guidelines and the Joint Commission on the Accreditation of Hospitals (JCAH) standards for medical record services do not.[11] Any hospital that is to be accredited by the JCAH must meet the standards defined in the *Accreditation Manual for Hospitals, 1986*. Any hospital that is to be reimbursed by the federal government must abide by the appropriate federal rules and regulations (Appendix 5–A). In addition, individual hospitals and physicians may offer guidelines for documentation to assist practitioners in developing adequate clinical documents (Appendix 5–B). These guidelines may be incorporated into the institution's Medical Staff bylaws.

In sum, the adequate patient record contains the data and the information selected by a group of professionals to best describe the health care experiences of provider and consumer. Through the use of carefully selected data elements, signs, and symbols, professionals with common understanding of appropriate use and meaning of language create a document that is useful to many groups. The benefits of the adequate record may be found in its power to assist in the care of the sick and the maintenance of health for society.

NOTES

1. K. Waters and G.F. Murphy, *Medical Records in Health Care Information* (Rockville, Md.: Aspen Publishers, Inc., 1979), p. 95.

2. "Background Paper: Uniform Minimum Health Data Sets," Department of Health and Human Services, Health Information Policy Council, Subcommittee on Data Comparability Standards (1983), pp. 1–23.

3. "Uniform Hospital Abstract—Minimum Basic Data Set," U.S. Department of Health, Education, and Welfare, U.S. National Committee on Vital and Health Statistics. DHEW Publication No.(HRA)75 1493 (Washington: Government Printing Office, 1972).

4. "Ambulatory Care Data: Report of the Conference on Ambulatory Care Records," Chicago, April 1972. Ed. Murnaghan (Philadelphia: J.H. Lippincott, 1973). (Reprinted from *Medical Care* 11(2): Supplement 1973).

5. "Long-Term Care Data: Report of the Conference on Long-Term Care Data," Tucson, May 1975. Ed. Murnaghan (Philadelphia: J.H. Lippincott, 1976). (Reprinted from *Medical Care* 14(5): Supplement, 1976).

6. "Background Paper: Uniform Minimum Health Data Sets," Department of Health and Human Services, Health Information Policy Council, Subcommittee on Data Comparability Standards (1983), p. 17.

7. "Background Paper: Uniform Minimum Health Data Sets," Department of Health and Human Services, Health Information Policy Council, Subcommittee on Data Comparability Standards (1983), p. 19.

8. P.B. Kritek, "Conceptual Considerations, Decision Criteria, and Guidelines Appropriate to the Development of a Nursing Minimum Data Set from a Practice Perspective." A commissioned paper for The Nursing Minimum Data Set Conference, May 15–16, 1985 (Milwaukee: University of Wisconsin, School of Nursing, 1985), p. 8.

9. Ibid.

10. K. Waters and G.F. Murphy, *Medical Records in Health Care Information* (Rockville, MD: Aspen Publishers, Inc., 1979), p. 65.

11. *Accreditation Manual for Hospitals, 1986* (Chicago: Joint Commission on the Accreditation of Hospitals, 1985), p. 87.

Appendix 5–A

Medical Record Service

PRINCIPLE

The hospital maintains medical records that are documented accurately and in a timely manner, are readily accessible, and permit prompt retrieval of information, including statistical data.

STANDARD I

An adequate medical record shall be maintained for each individual who is evaluated or treated as an inpatient, ambulatory care patient, or emergency patient, or who receives patient services in a hospital-administered home care program.

Interpretation

The purposes of the medical record are as follows:

—to serve as a basis for planning patient care and for continuity in the evaluation of the patient's condition and treatment;
—to furnish documentary evidence of the course of the patient's medical evaluation, treatment, and change in condition during the hospital stay, during an ambulatory care or emergency visit to the hospital, or while being followed in a hospital-administered home care program;
—to document communication between the practitioner responsible for the patient and any other health professional who contributes to the patient's care;

—to assist in protecting the legal interest of the patient, the hospital, and the practitioner responsible for the patient; and

—to provide data for use in continuing education and in research.

All significant clinical information pertaining to a patient is incorporated in the patient's medical record. The content of the medical record is sufficiently detailed and organized to enable

—the practitioner responsible for the patient to provide effective continuing care to the patient, determine later what the patient's condition was at a specific time, and review the diagnostic and therapeutic procedures performed and the patient's response to treatment;

—a consultant to render an opinion after an examination of the patient and a review of the medical record;

—another practitioner to assume the care of the patient at any time; and

—the retrieval of pertinent information required for utilization review and quality assurance activities.

To assure that the maximum possible information about any particular patient is available to the professional staff providing care, the unit record system is used. When it is not feasible to combine all inpatient, ambulatory care, and emergency records of an individual patient into a single unit record, a system is established to routinely assemble all divergently located record components when a patient is admitted to the hospital or appears for a prescheduled ambulatory care appointment; alternatively, there is a system that requires placing, in the ambulatory care or combined ambulatory care/emergency record file, copies of pertinent portions of each inpatient medical record, such as the discharge resume, the operative note, and the pathology report. Pertinent medical information obtained on request from outside sources is filed with, but not necessarily as part of, the patient's medical record. Such information is available to professional staff concerned with the care and treatment of the patient.

In the interest of facilitating the use of the medical record by all those authorized to review or make entries in it, as well as facilitating the retrieval of information for administrative, statistical, and quality assurance activities, it is recommended that a standardized format be developed for hospitalwide use. The format is approved by the medical staff through its designated mechanism. The use of a standardized format does not preclude making improvements in the medical record that will simplify the timely recording, review, or retrieval of information while not sacrificing the required content.

STANDARD II

The medical record contains sufficient information to identify the patient, support the diagnosis, justify the treatment, and document the results accurately.

Interpretation

Although the format and forms in use in the medical record will vary, all medical records contain the following:

—Identification data (when identification data are not obtainable, the reason is entered in the record)
—The medical history of the patient
—Reports of relevant physical examinations
—Diagnostic and therapeutic orders
—Evidence of appropriate informed consent (when consent is not obtainable, the reason is entered in the record)
—Clinical observations, including the results of therapy
—Reports of procedures, tests, and their results
—Conclusions at termination of hospitalization or evaluation/treatment

Inpatient medical records include at least the following:

—Identification data. These data include the patient's name, address, date of birth, and next of kin. There also is a number that identifies the patient and the patient's medical record(s).
—The medical history of the patient. The history includes the following information: the chief complaint; details of the present illness, including, when appropriate, assessment of the patient's emotional, behavioral, and social status; relevant past, social, and family histories; and an inventory by body systems. Whenever possible, the medical history is obtained from the patient. In programs for children and adolescents, an evaluation of developmental age factors and a consideration of educational needs are included, as appropriate. Opinions of the interviewer are not ordinarily recorded in the body of the history. The medical history is completed within the first 24 hours of admission to inpatient services. If a complete history has been obtained within a week prior to admission, such as in the office of a physician staff member or, when appropriate, the office of a qualified oral surgeon staff member, a durable, legible copy of this report may be used in the patient's hospital medical record, provided there have been no subsequent changes or the changes have been recorded at the time of admission. Obstetrical records include all prenatal information. A durable, legible original or reproduction of the office or clinic prenatal record is acceptable.
—The report of the physical examination. The report reflects a comprehensive, current physical assessment. The physical assessment is completed within the first 24 hours of admission to inpatient services. If a complete physical examination has been performed within a week prior to admission, such as in

the office of a physician staff member or, when appropriate, the office of a qualified oral surgeon staff member, a durable, legible copy of this report may be used in the patient's hospital medical record, provided there have been no changes subsequent to the original examination or the changes have been recorded at the time of admission. The recorded physical examination is authenticated by a physician or, when appropriate, by a qualified oral surgeon member of the medical staff. When a patient is readmitted within 30 days for the same or a related problem, an interval history and physical examination reflecting any subsequent changes may be used in the medical record, provided the original information is readily available, such as in a unit record. The medical record documents a current, thorough physical examination prior to the performance of surgery.

—A statement of the conclusions or impressions drawn from the admission history and physical examination. A statement of the course of action planned for the patient while in the hospital.

—Diagnostic and therapeutic orders. Such orders include those written by medical staff members, by physicians in training status, and by other individuals within the authority of their clinical privileges. Verbal orders of authorized individuals are accepted and transcribed by qualified personnel who are identified by title or category in the medical staff rules and regulations. The medical staff defines any category of diagnostic or therapeutic verbal orders associated with any potential hazard to the patient. Such orders are authenticated by the practitioner responsible for the patient within 24 hours.

—Evidence of appropriate informed consent. A policy on informed consent shall be developed by the medical staff and governing body and is consistent with any legal requirements. The medical record contains evidence of informed consent for procedures and treatments for which it is required by the policy on informed consent.

—Clinical observations.

    —Progress notes made by the medical staff. Progress notes give a pertinent chronological report of the patient's course in the hospital and reflect any change in condition and the results of treatment. Pertinent progress notes are also made by individuals so authorized by the medical staff, such as house staff members and individuals who have been granted clinical privileges.

    —Consultation reports. Each consultation report contains a written opinion by the consultant that reflects, when appropriate, an actual examination of the patient and the patient's medical record(s).

    —Nursing notes and entries by nonphysicians that contain pertinent, meaningful observations and information. When oxygen is prescribed for newborn infants, its use is recorded at least as an oxygen concentration percentage and at regular defined intervals, in accordance with a written policy of the newborn nursery. When there is a postanesthesia care unit, the medical record information includes the patient's level of consciousness on entering and leaving the unit, the patient's vital signs, and, when such are in use, the status of infusions, surgical dressings, tubes, catheters, and drains. Similar information is recorded in the medical records of patients whose postanesthesia recovery is accomplished in other than a special care unit.

—Opinions requiring medical judgment are written or authenticated only by medical staff members, house staff members, and other individuals who have been granted clinical privileges.

—Reports of procedures, tests, and their results. All diagnostic and therapeutic procedures are recorded and authenticated in the medical record. Any reports from facilities outside of the hospital may also be included, in which case the source facility is identified on the report.

—The individual who is responsible for the patient authenticates and records a preoperative diagnosis prior to surgery.

—Operative reports are dictated or written in the medical record immediately after surgery and contain a description of the findings, the technical procedures used, the specimens removed, the postoperative diagnosis, the name of the primary surgeon, and the names of any assistants. The completed operative report should be authenticated by the surgeon and filed in the medical record as soon as possible after surgery. When there is a transcription and/or filing delay, a comprehensive operative progress note is entered in the medical record immediately after surgery to provide pertinent information for use by any individual who is required to attend the patient.

—Reports of pathology and clinical laboratory examinations, radiology and nuclear medicine examinations or treatment, anesthesia records, and any other diagnostic or therapeutic procedures. Such reports are completed promptly and are filed in the record within 24 hours of completion, if possible.

—Medical records of donors and recipients of transplants. When an organ is obtained from a live donor for transplantation purposes, the medical records of the donor and recipient fulfill the requirements for any surgical inpatient medical record. When the donor organ is obtained from a brain-wave-death patient (where legally permissible), the medical record of the donor includes the date and time of brain-wave death, documentation by and identification of the physician who determined the death, the method of transfer of the organ, and the method of machine maintenance of the patient for organ donation, as well as an operative report. When a cadaver organ is removed for purposes of donation, there is an autopsy report that includes a description of the technique used to remove and prepare or preserve the donated organ. Reference should be made to pertinent state anatomical gift legislation for other medical record requirements.

—Conclusions at termination of hospitalization. Conclusions include the provisional diagnosis or reason(s) for admission, the principal and additional or associated diagnoses, the clinical resume or final progress note, and, when appropriate, the necropsy report.

—All relevant diagnoses established by the time of discharge, as well as all operative procedures performed, are recorded, using acceptable disease and operative terminology that includes topography and etiology as appropriate.

—The clinical resume concisely recapitulates the reason for hospitalization, the significant findings, the procedures performed and treatment rendered, the condition of the patient on discharge, and any specific instructions given to the patient and/or family, as pertinent. Consideration is given to instructions relating to physical activity, medication, diet, and follow-up care. The condition of the patient on discharge is stated in terms that permit a specific measurable comparison with the condition on admission, avoiding the use of vague relative terminology, such as "improved." When preprinted instructions are given to the patient or family, the record so indicates, and a sample of the instruction sheet in use at the time is on file in the medical record department. If authorized in writing by the patient or his legally qualified representative, a copy of the clinical resume is sent to any known medical practitioner and/or medical facility responsible for the subsequent medical care of the patient.

—A final progress note may be substituted for the resume in the case of patients with problems of a minor nature who require less than a 48-hour period of hospitalization and in the case of normal newborn infants and uncomplicated obstetrical deliveries. The final progress note includes any instructions given to the patient and/or family.

—In the event of death, a summation statement is added to the record either as a final progress note or as a separate resume. The final note indicates the reason for admission, the findings and course in the hospital, and the events leading to death.

—When a necropsy is performed, provisional anatomic diagnoses are recorded in the medical record within three days, and the complete protocol is made part of the record within 90 days.

STANDARD III

Medical records are confidential, secure, current, authenticated, legible, and complete.

The quality of the medical record depends in part on the timeliness, meaningfulness, authentication, and legibility of the informational content. Entries in medical records are made only by individuals given this right as specified in hospital and medical staff policies. All entries in the record are dated and authenticated, and a method is established to identify the authors of entries. Identification may include written signatures, initials, or computer key. When rubber stamp signatures are authorized, the individual whose signature the stamp represents places in the administrative offices of the hospital a signed statement to the effect that he or she is the only one who has the stamp and is the only one who will use it. There is no delegation of the use of such a stamp to another individual. The parts of the medical record that are the responsibility of the medical practitioner are authenticated by him or her. For example, when nonphysicians have been approved for such duties as taking medical histories and documenting some aspects of a physical examination, such information is appropriately authenticated by the physician responsible for the patient. When members of the house staff are involved in patient care, sufficient evidence is documented in the medical record to substantiate the active participation in, and supervision of, the patient's care by the attending physician responsible for the patient. Any entries in the medical record by house staff or nonphysicians that require countersigning by supervisory or attending medical staff members are defined in the medical staff rules and regulations.

To avoid misinterpretation, symbols and abbreviations may be used in the medical record only when they have been approved by the medical staff and when there is an explanatory legend available to those authorized to make entries in the medical record and to those who must interpret them. Each abbreviation or symbol has only one meaning.

In the interest of accuracy, legibility, and responsibility, and when budgetary and personnel availability permit, medical record entries, when appropriate, are typed. Special consideration is given to the typing of radiology and pathology reports, operative reports, and clinical resumes. When transcription and filing of these medical record reports cannot be accomplished in a timely manner, written entries pertinent to the continuity of the patient care shall be recorded.

Each clinical event, including the history and physical examination, is documented as soon as possible after its occurrence. The records of discharged patients are completed within a period of time that in no event exceeds 30 days following discharge. The period of time is specified in the medical staff rules and regulations. A medical record is ordinarily considered complete when the required contents, including any required clinical resume or final progress note, are assembled and authenticated, and when all final diagnoses and any complications are recorded, without use of symbols or abbreviations. Completeness implies that the content of any dictated record content has been transcribed and inserted into the medical record.

Source: Reprinted from *Accreditation Manual for Hospitals, 1986*, pp. 87–95, with permission of the Joint Commission on the Accreditation of Hospitals, © 1985.

Appendix 5–B

Sample Guidelines for Preparing Records

INTRODUCTION

Historically, the patient medical record has been used to provide accurate, timely information about the patient's condition and treatment. In recent years, the information in the medical record has become important to fiscal reimbursement. Documentation of patient care delivered under the Prospective Payment System, utilizing Diagnosis Related Groups (DRGs) as the basis for payment, requires even greater emphasis on accuracy and completeness of documentation.

PROFESSIONAL REVIEW ORGANIZATION OF WASHINGTON

The Social Security Amendments of 1983 established a Prospective Payment System for Medicare and specified that a Professional Review Organization (PRO) must review: the validity of diagnostic and procedural information supplied by the provider; the completeness and adequacy of the quality of care provided; *the appropriateness of admission and discharges*; and the medical necessity for which payment is sought when costs significantly exceed DRG prospective payment rates. Based on the results of its review, PRO determines whether payment should be made for services provided.

The only source of information to the PRO in making this determination is the patient medical record.

PRO surveyors review medical records to validate DRG designation upon which reimbursement is based. Surveyors also:

- *Review admissions for medical necessity*—The physician's medical record documentation must support hospital admission. Admission orders must reflect immediate need for acute level of care. If the admission is not justified, payment for the entire stay will be denied.

103

- *Review transfers to psychiatric and rehabilitation units exempt from PPS*—The physician's medical record documentation must justify continued stay throughout the hospital course, or "unnecessary days" will be denied (even if in the middle of the stay).
- *Review 100 percent pacemaker insertion procedures*—The physician's medical record documentation must justify the appropriateness and necessity of pacemaker insertion.
- *Review day outliers*—(lengths of stay that exceed the DRG's average length of stay by a specific amount)—The physician's medical record documentation must justify continued stay throughout the hospital course, or "unnecessary days" will be denied (even if in the middle of the stay).
- *Review cost outliers*—(exceed DRG costs by a specific amount although not a length of stay or day outlier)—The physician's medical record documentation must indicate all services rendered were medically necessary and appropriate.
- *Review readmissions within seven days of discharge from an acute care facility*—The PRO will review to determine whether:

—the two confinements are related;
—if not related, the second admission is medically necessary and appropriate;
—the patient was discharged prematurely from the first hospitalization.

- *Validate DRGs*—The PRO must verify that the diagnostic and procedural information that led to the DRG assignment is substantiated by the physician's documentation in the medical record.

DEFINITIONS OF TERMS

The following are UHDDS (Uniform Hospital Discharge Data Set) and federal definitions. These should be used when completing the record.

- *Principal Diagnosis*—The condition established *after study* to be chiefly responsible for the admission of the patient to the hospital. Place first on discharge sheet.
- *Other Diagnoses*—All conditions that exist at the time of admission that affect the treatment received and/or length of stay. Old diagnoses that relate to an earlier episode and have no bearing on this hospital stay are to be *excluded*.
- *Complications/Comorbidities (CCo)*

—*Complications*—All conditions that develop *after* the admission that affect treatment received and/or length of stay

—*Comorbidity*—A significant condition that exists upon admission that affects the treatment received and/or length of stay

- *Procedure*—A significant procedure is one that carries an operative or anesthetic risk, requires highly trained personnel, or requires special facilities or equipment. When more than one procedure is performed, the following criteria are used in determining the *principal procedure:* (1) one that was performed for definitive treatment rather than one performed for diagnostic or exploratory purposes, or was necessary to take care of a complication; (2) one that is most related to the principal diagnoses. To assure uniform reporting of significant procedures, ICD-9-CM codes are grouped into four classes (these groupings are published separately in UHDDS Classes of Procedures, ICD-9-CM CPHA, September 1978, Ann Arbor, Mich.) In general, Class I represents "surgery." Classes II and III correspond to other "significant procedures." Class IV represents other procedures and most of these codes are not significant for reporting purposes.

GUIDELINES AND EXAMPLES FOR PHYSICIANS

- *Use approved, specific medical terminology*
- *Provide complete information:*
  - —Document admitting diagnosis.
  - —Provide evidence in writing that the treatment is best provided on an inpatient basis.
  - —Document any condition that may affect utilization of resources.
  - —Provide documentation of all comorbidities and complications arising during the hospitalization.
  - —Document *all* diagnostic and therapeutic procedures on discharge sheet.
  - —Sign off on final diagnosis and procedures.
  - —Physician assuming responsibility as attending or discharging physician should document *all* diagnoses and procedures (not just those relating to his/her specialty) before signing off.
  - —Provide documentation to support final diagnosis and procedures at time of discharge.
- *Record a diagnosis, and not an operative procedure, as the principal diagnosis.*
  - Correct: Principal Diagnosis—herniated nucleus pulposis
  -             Procedure—laminectomy
  - Incorrect: Laminectomy
- *The admitting diagnosis or chief complaint should not necessarily be listed as the principal diagnosis.*

- *"Rule Out," R/O, and "Ruled Out"*

  —When the terms "Ruled Out" or R/O appear at the *beginning* of a diagnostic statement, it is treated as a suspected condition that is to be *ruled out*, such as R/O duodenal ulcer, 532.90. The code may be used as a principal diagnosis if the suspected condition was the chief reason, after study, occasioning the admission.

  —When the term "ruled out" or R/O appears at the *end* of a diagnostic statement, it is treated as no evidence of a specific condition found and the appropriate V code is assigned, such as "duodenal ulcer, ruled out," V71.8. The V code may be used as the principal diagnosis code if the suspected condition was the chief reason for the admission or encounter. For example:

	Incorrect	*Correct*
Principal Diagnosis:	Rule Out MI	Angina Pectoris
DRG:	143	140
DRG Wt:	.6814	.7548

- *Other Hints to Provide Specific Diagnoses*
  Specify:

  Acute/Chronic: List acute condition as principal diagnosis
  —Acute and Chronic, use Acute bronchitis
  —Acute, use Acute
  —Chronic, would not be used as principal
  Adverse Effect of a Correct Substance Properly Administered:
  —Manifestation
  —Drug
  Asthma
  —Status asthmaticus (if applicable)
  Burn
  —Degree
  —Site
  Complications
  —Cause
  Diabetes Mellitus
  —Insulin dependent
  —Noninsulin dependent
  Fracture
  —Closed or open
  —Specific anatomical site

Hypertension
—Benign or malignant
—With heart condition, specify if the heart condition is "due to" hypertension

Late Effect of an Injury (residual)
—Type of late injury
—Cause

Neoplasms
—For all neoplasms, specify which part of the organ is affected. For example:

Lung:	Breast:
upper lobe	upper inner quadrant
lower lobe	lower inner quadrant
middle lobe	upper outer quadrant
carena	lower outer quadrant
hilus	axillary tail

—Leukemia, Lymphoma, specify in remission
    Lymphosarcoma and reticulosarcoma
    Hodgkin's Disease
—Other malignant neoplasms of lymphoid and histiocytic tissue, specify
    Lymph nodes of head, face, and neck
    Intrathoracic lymph nodes
    Intraabdominal lymph nodes
    Lymph nodes of axilla and upper limb
    Lymph nodes of inguinal region and lower limb
    Intrapelvic lymph nodes
    Spleen
    Lymph nodes of multiple sites

Metastatic
—Primary site
—Is primary site still present or resected?
—Metastatic from _____ to _____
    If a primary site was removed on a previous hospitalization and there is no recurrence of the original site, list as the principal diagnosis the metastatic site if one exists. List the history of the primary as the secondary diagnosis. If a primary site was removed during the current hospitalization, list the primary site as the principal diagnosis and any metastatic sites as secondary diagnoses.

If patient is admitted for chemotherapy, use the following phrase: "Admitted for chemotherapy" (type of cancer, site, metastatic or primary).

Newborns
—List on the Newborn Discharge Summary all conditions present; e.g., jaundice
—List the cause of any condition, e.g., ABO incompatibility, jaundice

OB
—Antepartum, intrapartum, postpartum condition
—Indications for C-section, forceps, all procedures

Organisms (in infection)
—For example, *E. coli*

Poisoning Agent
—Drugs given in error, suicide, homicide, adverse effects when taken in combination with alcohol, or self-prescribed medications
　Specify poisoning
　Specify drug

Source: Courtesy of St. Joseph's Hospital, St. Paul, Minn. and Group Health Central Hospital, Seattle, Wash.

Chapter 6

A Mandate for Group Practice

Mary Alice Krill

The group practice form of medicine has long been believed to foster efficiency of medical services delivery. This chapter examines the reasons for this belief, first by describing the history of group practice and its rationale, then discussing pressures in the existing environment that have inflated costs, and finally examining the inherent capacity of medical groups to resist these pressures in an era of uncertainty.

Concern over the cost of medical care is not new. In 1932, a Senate subcommittee investigating the high cost of medical care recommended the establishment of group practices so that economies of medical personnel and medical costs could be realized.[1] Even so, for many years group practice physicians were looked upon by their peers as potential socialists who were courting government favor. The government's early stamp of approval indirectly promoted organized medicine's drastic censure of practices, and it was only after World War II that group practice began to be recognized.

By 1958 the climate had changed, with the American Medical Association urging a more tolerant attitude toward group physicians. In 1967 the AMA sponsored the First National Congress on Socioeconomics of Health Care.[2] The Congress promoted the positive aspects of group practice, such as efficiency and quality of care. That same year the Department of Health, Education, and Welfare (DHEW) initiated a national conference on group practice.[3] The conference recommended that government encourage the use of group practice under Medicare and Medicaid as a means of enhancing quality control.

In 1969 the IRS began to allow professionals to operate under incorporation, thus permitting physicians to benefit from corporate status, especially in regard to taxable current income. Over the five years following the Health Maintenance Organization Act of 1973, DHEW spent a total of $375 million to stimulate interest in the group model concept. Unfortunately, earlier constraints imposed through regulation greatly limited the impact of the act. Later legislative changes eliminated most of these requirements.

The flurry of HMO activity in the early 1980s reflected changes in their requirements for federal qualification and in pressures from government and consumers to moderate costs. InterStudy's annual HMO census estimated that enrollment in HMOs increased by 22.4 percent to 16,742,630 between December 1983 and December 1984. Under the Tax Equity and Fiscal Responsibility Act (TEFRA) of 1982, HMOs gained the right to enroll Medicare beneficiaries on a capitated basis, providing both Part A and Part B services. By June of 1985, 180 plans were enrolling Medicare members. Almost 5 percent of the total enrolled were Medicare beneficiaries.[4]

GROWTH OF GROUP PRACTICE

Tracing the roots of medical group practice in this country provides an insight to its rationale. Medical knowledge exploded at the turn of the century, sending physicians into more highly differentiated specialties. Patient care was fragmented and concern for the whole patient was lost sight of by those rushing toward esoteric forms of practice. Only by bringing these specialists together to practice medicine at one site would patient continuity of care be assured. Group practice pioneers, from Mayo and Johns Hopkins, trained other physicians who took their forms of practice across the country, starting new multispecialty group practices. In those days as now, physicians joined groups in order to provide specialty facilities beyond the reach of solo practice.

The number of physicians in medical groups as well as the number of such groups grew steadily, resulting in the greatest concentration of these entities in states last admitted to the Union and in those with the smallest population densities. Both the AMA (in 1965, 1969, 1975, and 1980) and the U.S. Public Health Service (1946 and 1959) have collected information on medical groups.

The AMA and the Medical Group Management Association (MGMA) agree upon the definition of a medical group practice: a formally organized group of at least three licensed physicians who are engaged in the practice of medicine as a legally recognized entity, sharing business management, facilities, records, and personnel. Founded in 1926, the MGMA is the oldest and largest organization (6,000 individual and 2,800 medical group members) representing medical group practice. In 1973, MGMA established its research affiliate, the Center for Research in Ambulatory Health Care Administration (the Center for Research).

The number of group practice physicians as a percentage of total nonfederal patient care physicians rose from 16.2 percent in 1969 to 25.8 percent in 1980.[5] Data are not available on the extent of physician growth between 1980 and 1984. Although the number of physicians in groups has continued to increase, the overall average size of groups as measured by the number of full-time-equivalent physicians declined steadily between 1959 and 1969. This change reflected the formation of many more single-specialty groups, which tend to be small. From 1969 through 1975 this trend was reversed, and average group size increased, indicating more physicians were joining existing groups. Between 1975 and 1980, groups of five or fewer physicians increased at almost twice the rate of larger groups. Further, according to a *Medical Economics* study, even in 1972 at least 50 percent of all physicians did not consider themselves to be in solo practice but rather engaged in some type of shared arrangements with others.

In 1969, single-specialty groups comprised 50 percent of all groups; in 1984 they represented 70 percent, growing 235.6 percent since 1969. The AMA's 1985 publication on medical groups shows 140,392 nonfederal physician positions in 15,485 groups.[5] Multispecialty groups were 18.3 percent of the total in 1984. As a percentage of total groups, this number had dropped from 38.0 percent in 1969. The number of physicians practicing in multispecialty groups, however, was more than the total in single specialties. That number is continuing to grow, from an average size of 10.1 physicians in 1969 to 26.6 in 1984.

The MGMA's 2,800 member groups average about 28 FTE physicians in 1986, up from 14 in 1975; however, median size group is 7. These groups are both multispecialty and single specialty, with 48 separate specialties identified in MGMA's data base. It is very probable that the growth in numbers and sizes of medical groups represents a continuing response to market forces. New physicians enter groups, have ready access to patients, guaranteed income, and yet are able to enjoy a quality of life that comes with covered time off and predictable hours. According to Freshnock and Jensen, small groups may be more palatable to physicians in the beginning because of their wish to maintain a degree of independence yet respond to market forces.[6] As time goes on, large groups may be more attractive because they have bigger patient bases and are financially more stable.

THE CHALLENGE FOR MEDICAL GROUPS

In the past medical groups were relatively free from regulation, but that situation appears to be changing rapidly. Despite the Reagan Administration's preference for fostering competition, the government, as the largest purchaser of medical services, cannot ignore the $1 billion a day spent on health care in the United States. One of the significant factors in reducing cost is to limit or provide a substitute for the most expensive component of care—services provided in the hospital. It has been generally assumed that the logical and less expensive alternative is ambulatory care, shifting many medical services to the outpatient sector. In the meantime, data are being sought to substantiate this assumption, which may be in dispute. Thus the challenge for medical groups of necessity includes the following:

- Quality of care must be maintained according to agreed-upon standards.
- Cost of care must be competitive and affordable.
- Care must be accessible.
- A broad range of services must be available.
- Care must be delivered effectively and efficiently.
- Incentives for cost moderation must exist for providers, consumers, and any third party payers involved.
- Business and industry requirements must be fulfilled.
- Alternative delivery mechanisms must be included.
- Physician needs must be met.

EXTERNAL PRESSURES ON MEDICAL GROUPS

All system objectives of a group practice through which its mission is accomplished are influenced to a significant degree by pressures from a variety of outside sources. Figure 6–1 depicts four primary external forces that affect a medical group's capability for competing—the environment, regulations, medical technology, and incentives. Exploration of each one of these elements in more detail can provide an understanding of the expectations for their control. Medical groups' inherent capacities for developing internal strategies to manage their destinies indicate how they can meet these mounting pressures.

According to University of Colorado futurist Leland R. Kaiser, strategic planning for medical groups must encompass four features: the economic, demographic, social, and political forecasts of the service area.[7] Future realities for medical groups should be envisioned in terms of the impact of the following predictions.

Figure 6–1 External Forces in Group Practice

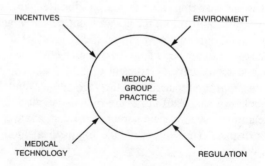

The Competitive Environment

The most pervasive external influence to have an impact on the medical group is its immediate environment. Pressures from government to increase consumers' knowledge of medical care opportunities parallel the groups' need to maintain their market share in an increasingly competitive climate. While some groups have adopted a reactive stance to competition and subsequently have watched their presence in the community diminish, others are proactive in their responses. New services being offered by these latter providers include patient education programs, occupational medicine specialties, gerontology outreach programs and home health services, and prepaid medical services (by affiliation with HMOs or by setting up their own plans).

These same groups are in the forefront of attempts to gain industry's attention and to negotiate competitive capitation rates for expanded services, including preventive care and health status assessments. Examples are participation in preferred provider organizations (PPOs), industrial self-insurance plans, and other medical service contracts. Brushed by the reality of physician oversupply, medical groups are finding it necessary to market for survival. Administrators in turn are attempting to convince their groups that in the future only productive, efficient providers will attract patients. It is anticipated that provider contracts in the future will be based on services and efficiency as well as on price discounts. Expanded coverage offered by medical groups to Medicare beneficiaries under risk contracts seems to bear this out. Continuing consumer demand for increased services undoubtedly will moderate extensive discounting.

There is a longevity revolution in America. Group practices with 30 percent of their business represented by care of the elderly are in a good position to extend the management of their care to a comprehensive case management continuum. In this model, the medical groups would coordinate the care of the elderly, ranging from preventive and health maintenance activities such as aerobics and smoking cessation to home care, functional assessments, and rehabilitation. Implementing such a model would require medical groups to network and joint-venture with other community agencies so that the social, medical, health education, and recreational needs of the elderly can be met in a cost-effective way. The economies of scale, the scope of services, and the information systems in place in medical groups have tremendous implications for cost benefits to the increasing numbers of aged. Further, the case-mix management system (see Case-Mix Management Software, page 210) developed by the Center for Research would allow medical groups to establish resource consumption profiles for different categories of elderly such as age 65 to 75, 75 to 85, or 85 and older. Comparative data and trend analyses could then measure the effects of certain programs, for example health maintenance, on the health status of specific elderly populations.

Market forces are accounting for dramatic changes in the structure of the health industry. Large, integrated medical firms are emerging. Hospital Corporation of America (HCA) and American Medical International (AMI) are multinational organizations that can provide marketing expertise and additional economies of scale, as well as infuse capital into medical groups. Often these groups own small hospitals and the national firms can engage in a variety of joint ventures that are profitable for all parties. The relationships of the Lovelace Foundation in Albuquerque with HCA and the Scripps Foundation in La Jolla with HCA are two examples. The prestigious Mayo Clinic has expanded its services by purchasing hospitals, by entering the HMO business, and by setting up satellite group practices in Arizona and Florida.

The new bottom line as far as consumers are concerned is the amount of "health produced per dollar spent." The control mechanisms being perfected by HMOs, particularly in regard to utilization patterns, are the most effective techniques available for cost moderation, thus the government interest in promoting capitation arrangements. However, development and maintenance of a sound competitive system are predicated on the existence of fair market choice, where most consumers are provided multiple choices by employers or by Medicare and Medicaid. Unfortunately, many areas of the country are served only by one or two provider organizations.

Many medical groups are becoming integrated vertically (embracing several levels of care) and horizontally (forging relationships with other ambulatory care organizations) with other provider entities. Of the MGMA member groups, 132 are academic practices associated with medical schools and teaching hospitals. Many groups are sharing services or forming more formal liaisons such as the fee-for-service/prepaid groups and PPOs comprising Preferred Providers of America in California. This umbrella organization provides management expertise to groups by contracting with PPOs, which in turn provide marketing and administrative services on behalf of the member groups. Large multispecialty groups are setting up or acquiring primary care groups, ambulatory surgery units, and long-term care facilities.

The Role of Regulation

A second major pressure comes from state and federal legislative and regulatory actions. The increasing involvement of state governments is predicted. Regulations on private business, such as the Employee Retirement Income Security Act of 1974 (ERISA), the Economic Recovery and Tax Act of 1981 (ERTA), and the Tax Equity and Fiscal Responsibility Act of 1982 (TEFRA) have indirectly affected the choice of legal organizational structures. Coupled with the advent of professional corporations and their accompanying tax benefits, efficiency of governance, and reduced liability, these regulations have influenced the choice of legal form that has evolved for medical groups: statistics from the AMA indicate that 73 percent of all medical groups now are corporations, outstripping partnerships by five to one.

In the past, reimbursement policies appeared to discriminate against ambulatory care, with higher payments to physicians for performing procedures in inpatient settings. Group practices often were reimbursed for considerably less than the costs of treatment. New techniques for data accumulation, retrieval, analysis, and reporting now are making it possible for medical groups to provide government and other payers with the hard facts of the costs of delivering outpatient care. With the administration's emphasis on free-market competition, studies focusing on comparisons among different medical practice patterns assume a new importance.

The Health Care Financing Administration (HCFA), for example, has been interested in studies aimed at demonstrating new physician payment arrangements for services to Medicare beneficiaries such as risk contracts with HMOs, direct physician capitation, payment based on ambulatory visit groups (prospective pricing for outpatient services), and payment for physicians' services in the hospital based on diagnosis related groups (DRGs). Demonstrations of risk contracting with HMOs for the treatment of Medicare patients have been completed with funding by HCFA and now more than 70 HMOs are engaged in risk contracting. The risk contract concept is a part of most HMO operations. The HMO receives a predetermined or capitated amount for each individual enrolled and provides a set of covered benefits, regardless of the cost of actually providing them. Demonstrations of direct physician capitation under Medicare also are anticipated.

The Impact of Medical Technology

Just as computer technology has evolved into high-capacity, lower cost equipment, so has medical technology, resulting in less expensive, less complex procedures, safely performed in an outpatient setting. A third external force that is affecting groups is medical technology. New forms and methods of treatment are placing hospitals in a position similar to that of the mainframe computer. First-dollar coverage insurance programs, limited to care in hospitals, are ineffectual.

New types of insurance plans that offer incentives for cost savings involve prepayment, self-insurance, copayments, coordination of benefits, and other arrangements. Benefits are changing and ambulatory surgery is becoming commonplace. Disincentives for cost savings inherent in total coverage insurance plans gradually are being eroded. Many large medical groups have incorporated ambulatory surgery centers into their facilities. Together with a focus on preventive care and wellness, cost savings have inured to the benefit of consumers.

The Creation of Incentives for Cost Control

The last element to be discussed is the challenge of creating appropriate incentives for controlling costs in a medical group. Health care expenditures in 1984 comprised 10.6 percent of the gross national product, or one billion per day, and are expected to reach 12 percent in 1990. Although physician fees account for less than 20 percent of those costs, physicians are said to be responsible for a significant amount of other charges by virtue of tests and procedures they order. They also control patients' admissions into hospitals and their lengths of stay.

According to a General Accounting Office study, physicians directly control or influence 70 percent of the dollars spent for health care. Incentives inherent in prepayment arrangements that put the physicians at risk for unnecessary hospital stays, for referred treatments, and for extraneous tests and procedures have been shown to have the effect of lowering the costs controlled by physicians. The techniques discussed below are employed by prepaid medical groups affiliated with HMOs.

The most effective controls resulting in cost-beneficial physician performance occur in group model HMOs. Existing fee-for-service medical groups often convert a portion of their operation to prepaid practice. These groups already are established in facilities, have peer review mechanisms in place, and have the ability to accumulate and retrieve information on patient mix and treatment, so that prepaid components initiated by existing fee-for-service groups have a high probability of success.

In addition, practice patterns established under the prepayment component appear to influence fee-for-service delivery effectiveness. A study by St. Louis Park Medical Center (now merged with the Nicolett Clinic to form the Park Nicolett Medical Center), comparing its fee-for-service with its prepaid practice, supports this contention. At the time of the study, the fee-for-service and prepaid practice percentages of total business were approximately equal.[8]

The independent practice association (IPA), another form of HMO that coordinates prepaid care by fee-for-service solo practitioners and by fee-for-service group physicians, has been more acceptable to traditional providers. However, solo physicians engaged in prepayment alternatives through contracts with IPAs are less apt to change their medical practice patterns. Because only a small percentage of their income is derived from treating HMO patients, they are inclined to perpetuate less efficient activities than are group practice physicians who combine prepaid and fee-for-service medicine. However, some fee-for-service-only medical groups, such as the Mayo Clinic, are able to operate at costs comparable to the most successful HMOs. (See Nobrega et al., 1979.)

Other medical staff incentives involve the relationship of physician income and productivity. More efficient use of doctors' time through the scheduling and use of physician extenders and other allied health personnel results in time and money savings that can be passed on to patients. A characteristic of multispecialty groups that greatly influences cost is their ability to match specialties and facilities to their patient populations. In the future, the groups that can control expenses will survive because they will be able to compete in terms of cost to the purchasers of health care services.

ORGANIZATIONAL STRUCTURES AND RESPONSES

As for the internal responses being made by medical groups, it is helpful to examine their organizational structures and the management techniques available to them. Figure 6–2 emphasizes the advantages inherent in medical groups and the tools and techniques immediately accessible for containing costs. While the efficiency of HMOs has been attributed primarily to incentives produced by prepayment, it is thought that the organization and structure of group practices may be an equally strong predictor of the group model HMO's efficiency.

Inherent Advantages in Groups

A successful medical group is able to combine separate but functionally interrelated health care delivery components into a unified whole. This cohesiveness is possible because the group is a defined system for delivering efficient, effective health care.

The very reasons that make group practice enticing to physicians also place medical groups in the best position to moderate spiraling costs and to compete. Earlier it was noted that the advantages to the physicians in this type of practice are greater efficiency, economy, and professional benefits, especially to those entering practice.

Figure 6–2 Internal Forces Affecting Group Practice

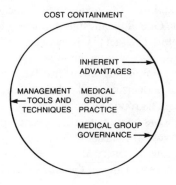

All things considered, the two most important advantages of groups are (1) the benefits to be realized from economies of scale and (2) the capability of extending the scope of services offered beyond the capacity of solo practice. Earlier studies[9] have suggested that the optimal scale occurs at a relatively small practice size. Jeff Goldsmith, a business consultant, supports this view. Annual cost surveys of the MGMA membership for the periods 1978-1985, however, show this trend to be multimodal, with economies increasing at intervals as groups grow larger. Further, the ability to provide unified medical record systems, utilization and medical audit reviews, and sophisticated budget planning, marketing, and control is better developed in larger groups.

In summary, then, three general characteristics of group practices seem to help ensure their effectiveness:

1. Success patterns for medical groups appear to be highly dependent upon the ability to maintain a unified medical record system.
2. The opportunity for colleagues to observe one another's work represents a natural advantage for maintaining quality through systematic peer review within the organized setting of the group.
3. The ability of group practice physicians to subordinate their own personal goals to those of the overall group contributes enormously to the group's future success.

Medical Group Governance

The governance of medical groups in many instances is similar to that of any small business enterprise. In one important respect, however, it differs from most businesses and from other health care delivery organizations; that is, the physicians generally fill two roles, that of owner or principal shareholder and that of primary operator and producer. A Center for Research study in 1979 investigated the roles of group practice administrators, medical directors, and governing bodies.[10] The report delineates responsibility and involvement of these three administrative echelons and lists 141 major tasks associated with conducting the medical group's business. One of the most important positions in the management team is that of administrator. The fact that someone is designated to be responsible for their business aspects gives groups an edge over solo practitioners. Study results show professional administrators to be involved with almost every management task, influencing major decisions and policy making through negotiation and persuasion. A 1983 survey on group practice governance and 1986 interviews with physicians and administrators confirm these roles are virtually unchanged.

When asked in the survey what tasks were considered critical, administrators overall identified "managing/reporting the financial status of the group" as the single most important. Characteristics of the medical group have an impact on the extent and importance of the administrator's tasks. The competitive environment tends to require that administrators be more involved in the external relations of the practice. This function is particularly relevant when the group has a significant amount of prepayment.

If medical groups are to compete in a dynamic marketplace, the physician/administrative team must adopt new strategies based on improved financial and productivity data regarding the practice. It may be important for groups to redefine their product lines based upon case mix much in the way hospitals have done based on DRGs. Medical groups typically have examined services such as radiology and laboratory and evaluated their fees and charges.

Medical groups are finding themselves under contract to treat new populations of individuals without much knowledge of the financial implications. Prepayment for some services and discounted fees for others put groups in the position of limiting their flow of revenue. Thus they must formulate new strategies for reducing the flow of funds out of the group. This can be done only by instilling in the group an understanding of cost behavior as opposed to charges.

Prospective pricing and prepayment are predicted to increase because these methods have the potential for improving utilization of resources and containing costs. Management decisions will have an effect on physician staffing, resource utilization, quality assurance, risk management, facilities management, financing, and marketing. Of necessity, information systems must be structured to capture and integrate clinical and financial information.

Physicians are knowledgeable and comfortable about choices regarding the clinical aspects of their practice but are less so concerning the financial aspects. It is imperative, therefore, that physicians and administrators work together as a team in making decisions on new strategies for retaining and improving market share.

Focusing on cost behavior may require some degree of decentralizing control. Costs are best controlled at the point of incurrence, usually the department level. The information system must provide clinical/financial data to individual physicians, department heads, satellites, and the group as a whole. Role definitions within the group will change as it experiences joint venturing, shared service agreements, contract negotiations, and possibly horizontal and vertical mergers.

The group's method for selecting and briefing of board members, board chairs, and medical directors will take on new importance. Administrators will have responsibility for continuing environmental assessments, including community plans and potential competition from new HMOs and PPOs. The aging of the population and the expectations for changes in Medicare reimbursement also must be considered. Constraints within the group organizational structure that preclude team building must be examined.

Groups whose physicians have high allegiance to the entity will be in the best position to thrive. Physicians will need to cooperate with one another and decisions will be needed on income distribution and retained earnings. Internal dissension could spell disaster. An example would be unrealistic needs by one or more physicians for autonomy and independence, resulting in refusal to subordinate individual goals to group goals. Groups with no equity also will be at a disadvantage when it is necessary to launch new programs in response to community needs. Access to additional capital may come from mergers and acquisitions. Hospitals and others will be competing for the outpatient business. Thus groups will need to determine a good match between the type and amount of information collected and the cost of collecting it. They also will need to define protocols for establishing and staffing review committees.

Medical records departments must be willing to set standards for the quality and type of information included in the records. Coding of procedures and diagnoses will need to be accurate and timely, with well-defined procedures for entering key data elements into the information system. The role of the management information service must be results oriented.

It may be expedient for the group to instigate patient education regarding use of the health care system. Patient demand for expensive but unnecessary treatment modalities drives up the cost per visit. This is of special concern with prepaid patients. Education and emphasis on preventive measures often can ameliorate such demands.

Medical groups thus must be aware of existing products and define new product lines. In doing so they must develop and nurture the administrative/physician team. The basis for the teams' decisions will be information generated by an integrated clinical and financial information system.

New Management Technology

A number of important management tools and techniques have been developed by MGMA's Center for Research, specifically for use in medical groups. Soulier and DeCoster, in a 1982 article on "Productivity versus Cost Control," noted that financial management systems in health care organizations had at best been custodial in nature.[11] *Practical Financial Management for Medical Groups* (1979), *Management Accounting for Health Maintenance Organizations* (1984), and *Management Accounting for Fee-for-Service/Prepaid Medical Groups* (1985), published by the Center, have helped dispel the custodial view and have contributed significantly to developing the new financial management technology needed. These systems, produced with funding from the W.K. Kellogg Foundation, can generate data to assist in briefing physician boards on the cost implications of their practice preferences. The texts include charts of accounts for medical groups and HMO plans that are incorporated into well-researched systems for budgeting, planning, and control.

Even in 1985, 36 percent of MGMA member groups indicated that they do not budget; 85 percent have no long-range plan; and 69 percent do not budget for capital equipment. Funding from The Robert Wood Johnson Foundation enabled the Center to establish and train a technical assistance network of group practice administrators. These consultants, now the MGMA Consulting Service, include both physician and nonphysician administrators and comprise teams that contract to assist groups having management problems.

Many administrators are using increasingly sophisticated techniques such as flexible budgeting, cost accounting, short- and long-range forecasting, trend analysis, and the use of comparative information for prospective decision making to provide effective management of their medical groups. The mean and median data in MGMA annual survey reports constitute normative standards for comparative purposes. The reports structured in relation to the charts of accounts also are useful for briefing physicians on cost-containment measures. Administrators believe that physicians who are made aware of the cost impact of their decisions are amenable to change if quality of care is not jeopardized. A 1982 report from the General Accounting Office to the Secretary of Health and Human Services on physician training supports this point of view.

The MGMA Financial Management Committee aids the development and use of new management technology. It reviews all Center proposals, plans, and projects related to financial management. It supports efforts resulting in financial reporting systems that provide administrators and physicians with trend data to be compared internally over time and externally with other medical groups. Workshops and seminars focus on implementation of coordinated financial systems and techniques for analyzing and interpreting data output for decision-making purposes. With a well-organized administrative staff, medical groups can supply reliable information for reimbursement purposes.

MGMA and the Center have a number of services and resources available to group practice administrators for improving their management information systems. These are discussed below.

Annual Cost Survey

As part of its data base management activities, the Medical Group Management Association has obtained cost and revenue information from its members since the mid-1950s. Administrators can use these annual cost survey reports to compare their groups' revenue and expense data with the mean average and median data for all groups. Information is tabulated according to medical group size (number of FTE physicians); by section of the country (West, South, East, Midwest); and by multispecialty and single specialty, according to specialty.

Groups report revenue in gross fee-for-service charges and prepaid contract changes, subsequently broken down to total cash collections. Detailed expenses are reported on 75 nonphysician-related and 11 physician-related categories. Medical groups also provide information on accounts receivable. Average total nonphysician overhead expense is presented for all categories. About 500 medical groups respond to MGMA's annual cost survey and about half of these are multispecialty groups (see Table 6–1). The data reflect total revenue and expenses for multispecialty medical group practices for 1983, 1984, and 1985.[12] Trends can be observed over those three years, with the relationships among the percentages remaining relatively stable over time.

Standard Cost-Accounting System

Groups would like to be able to compare themselves on a department-by-department basis and include allocations of overhead. Because different methods of cost accounting are used, these comparisons are unreliable. In 1986, the Center for Research developed a standard cost-accounting system that could be superimposed on data submitted by the groups. Administrative and other overhead costs would be allocated systematically by each group to various departments, comparisons made, and the results used by the group's management.

Annual Production Survey

The MGMA annual production survey captures physician, personal service, production information in 38 physician specialties and nine allied health professional areas. Realizing the problems with using physician gross charges information as a productivity measure, the Center for Research directs respondents to designate whether charge data result exclusively from clinical practice or include charges resulting from ancillary services.

The productivity of physicians in medical groups generally is higher compared with those in other practice settings. Group physicians tend to be more productive and to employ more nonphysician personnel. Nurses and medical assistants, together with business and clerical personnel, perform many of the tasks assumed by solo practitioners, thus releasing group physicians for more complex medical procedures.

Group Practice Performance Evaluator

In 1983, MGMA and the Center offered medical groups a quarterly Group Practice Performance Evaluator (GPPE) data service, developed with funds from the W.K. Kellogg Foundation in cooperation with Hospital Administrative Services of the American Hospital Association.

The GPPE is an evaluation/comparison report compiled from data provided by subscribing medical groups. Indicators are computed for the current quarter, the

Table 6–1 Cost Surveys of Medical Groups

MEDICAL GROUP MANAGEMENT ASSOCIATION
Group Mean Revenue and Expenses 1982-1984, U.S., Multispecialty Groups

	1982	1983	1984
Mean Cash Collections per Physician	$247,700 (100.0%)	$265,718 (100.0%)	$277,776 (100.0%)
Expenses as a Percentage of Mean Cash Collections:			
Nonphysician Salaries and Benefits	25.0%	25.2%	25.3%
Radiology and Laboratory	4.9	4.9	4.7
Medical Supplies	2.6	2.8	3.0
Building/Occupancy and Furniture/Equipment	7.8	8.0	8.1
Insurance Premiums	2.0	2.2	2.3
Other Expenses	7.5	7.1	7.0
Total Overhead	49.8%	50.2%	50.4%
Accounts Receivable per Physician	$79,000	$79,144	$82,210
Number of Months Revenue in Accounts Receivable	4.1	3.6	4.0
Adjusted Collection Percentage	98.1%	93.8%	93.9%
Employees per Physician	3.9	3.8	3.8
Number of Respondents	286	259	214

Source: *The Cost and Production Survey Report*, Medical Group Management Association, 1983, 1984, 1985.

previous quarter, the same quarter of the prior year, and the average of the past four quarters' data. Information provided by the GPPE can be used to:

- supplement managerial resources
- make general assessments of patient services
- identify problems
- identify seasonal and performance trends over specified time periods
- maintain managerial control
- control and reduce costs
- make decisions pertaining to the addition and/or elimination of clinical specialties
- make decisions regarding the development and expansion or reduction of ancillary services and profit centers
- conduct short- and long-range planning
- evaluate fees in relation to financial and utilization factors.

The GPPE uses indicator values to accomplish these tasks. Indicator values are ratios derived by simple algebraic equations that convert input data from all participating groups to a common base to allow performance comparisons to be made. Each subscriber's report has two separate comparisons—to all other subscribers and to a selected peer group such as groups of the same single specialty or multispecialty groups of similar sizes. More than 120 indicators are computed, providing a detailed look at the group's:

- physician production
- overhead
- employee staffing
- financial performance.

The Group Practice Performance Evaluator is designed to provide the productivity and efficiency information needed in the changing environment of the 1980s. An example from a medical group's summary report appears in Table 6–2.

A group can participate in the GPPE by providing essential financial data (group cash collections, summarized group expenses); physician production (billings, number of outpatient encounters, hospital admissions); and group staffing data (number of FTE physicians and employees) on a quarterly basis. MGMA computes and mails GPPE output reports within three weeks of the data submission deadline. If a group cannot provide input data for a quarter, a report is compiled using available historic and external group data.

Table 6-2 Group Practice Performance Evaluator

Medical Center

	Current Qtr 3 1985	Internal Trend Qtr 2 1985	Internal Trend Qtr 3 1984	Avg Past 4 Qtrs	Budget Comparison Estimate Qtr 3	Variance	External Comparison Compare Group CG. 1 Median	Rank	N
General Group Performance									
General Utilization									
1. Outpatient Encounters per FTE Physician	1,032.16	1,189.14	858.17	1,168.64			996.65	18	40
2. Hospital Admissions per FTE Physician	10.71	14.25	134.03	54.64			46.67	32	33
3. New Patient Registrations per FTE Physician	45.69	57.75	60.00	64.00			79.30	32	35
Financial Performance									
4. Total Gross Charges	$2,453,085.00	$2,571,403.00	$2,057,392.00	$2,351,266.25			$2,310,704.50	21	44

All data that identify a specific participating medical group are confidential and are not released without written permission. MGMA issues aggregate information as long as it does not identify any specific participant.

Techniques for Managing Medical Groups

Under a grant from The Henry J. Kaiser Family Foundation, the Center has provided medical group administrators and physicians with the tools they need to diversify and expand their practices. In the increasingly competitive marketplace, fee-for-service medical groups are adding a prepaid component by affiliation with or forming HMOs. Meeting consumer demand for cost containment through close scrutiny of utilization, while emphasizing quality assurance, enables medical groups to provide their patients appropriate care at affordable costs. The *Going Prepaid* series of seven monographs published by the Center, and related educational seminars conducted by the Center, cover these topics: strategic planning, legal issues, management information systems, actuarial issues, marketing management, the role of the medical director, and evaluating the performance of a prepaid medical group.

Case-Mix Management Software

Under funding from the W.K. Kellogg Foundation, the Center conducted a demonstration in five medical groups to develop and test a case-mix methodology for evaluating utilization of services in a medical group over periods of time and in comparison to similar groups. The case-mix methodology is designed to measure, monitor, and assess the efficiency and effectiveness of physician care.

The project investigated several outpatient case-mix methodologies such as ambulatory visit groups (AVGs) and diagnosis clusters, together with a relative value scale in *Relative Values for Physicians,* published by McGraw-Hill in 1984. This research was finalized in software programs, designed for use on IBM personal or IBM-compatible computers to integrate a medical group's clinical and financial information. The case-mix system links physician production measured by physicians' Current Procedural Terminology, 4th ed. (CPT-4) procedures.[13] They are weighted by the relative value scale and matched with the presenting diagnosis to track the resulting physician resource consumption.

The system was tested initially at five medical group sites: Carle Clinic Association, Urbana, Ill.; the Mason Clinic/Virginia Mason Hospital, Seattle; the Mayo Clinic, Rochester, Minn.; Park Nicollet Medical Center, Minneapolis; and the University Park Medical Center, Denver. The tests sought to determine resource consumption internally and in comparison with other groups. The GPPE described earlier was used for the external comparisons. During the grant period, the system also was tested by smaller group practices, and in the postfunded period was to be made available to all parties in the health care field. Protocols and guides for implementing the case-mix measurement system were to be available to group practices and to ambulatory care centers, HMOs, and PPOs.

The first phase of the project, based on physician services described by CPT-4s, resulted in a software program, the Physician Procedures/Values Report, that enables administrators and medical directors to study group physicians' practice styles. This process can include generating reports that describe individual physicians' contributions to their departments and to the group as a whole in terms of procedures (CPT-4s), charges, and relative value units. Management decisions involving fees and financial risk can be made, based on productivity in fee-for-service practices and expense in prepaid practices respectively.

The case-mix measurement system, involving ICD-9 diagnosis data in addition to CPT-4s, charges, and relative value units, enables health care organizations to collect and analyze information on the utilization of medical services in response to given diagnoses. Such information then can be used to evaluate productivity changes and appropriateness of care as well as to predict resource consumption. The information also would be of value to consumers and the business community to aid them in choices of medical service delivery. The case-mix measurement system allows medical groups, either singly or in concert, to influence and be prepared for any legislation or regulations requiring physician services to be reimbursed based on Medicare prospective pricing or capitated risk contract programs.

Tools and technology resulting from the project include the following:

• Software and operations manual for implementing:

1. Physician Procedures/Values Report
2. case-mix management system

• Protocols for using case-mix data for:

1. strategic planning and budgeting
2. forecasting resource consumption
3. measuring physician productivity
4. describing physician practice patterns
5. designing income distribution plans

• Educational programs and articles on how to implement and how to use the systems and software produced by the project.

The Center for Research conducted and managed the project with the advice of the funder and a project advisory board/task force. The latter was formed to recommend and review processes and materials in the developmental stages.

Members of the advisory board and task force included physicians, administrators, management information directors, and medical records personnel—all in medical group practices.

ENCOURAGEMENT ON COSTS

The examples of the tools and techniques being developed for medical groups should be encouraging to consumers, government, and industry looking to such medical delivery organizations for an abatement in rising health care costs. As Paul Ellwood has stated, "Remarkably little is known about group practice . . . . Most importantly, each medical care organization needs a health care management information system and a balance sheet."[14] These are necessary "to quantify progress toward quality objectives."

The proportion of physicians under 35 years of age in groups is increasing (15.1 percent in 1980, up from 9.3 percent in 1975 according to the AMA). These figures seem to support new physicians' preferences to share administrative functions. Between 1969 and 1980, the number of physicians in groups more than doubled: In 1969 there were only 40,093; in 1980, 88,290; in 1984, 140,392 (this number may be somewhat inflated because physicians may be listed in more than one group but recognizes significant 1980-1984 growth). The average annual rate of growth in the number of medical groups increased from 4.9 percent in the periods 1969-1975 and 1975-1980 to 9.5 percent between 1980 and 1984.

Access to comprehensive care, economies of scale, organized administrative and medical records capacity, dynamics of peer review, and the ability to offer physician incentives—these factors are strengths that will make group practice the dominant presence in the future health care community.

NOTES

1. John E. Kralewski and Roice D. Luke, *Group Practice: Review and Recommendations for Planning and Research* (Chicago: Blue Cross and Blue Shield Associations, 1979), p. 3.

2. Commission on Medical Care Plans, *Journal of the American Medical Association* Special Edition (January 17,1959), p. 48.

3. U.S. Department of Health, Education, and Welfare, "Group Practice Pre-Payment Organization" (Washington, DC: HSMHA, March 29, 1970), pp. 1–9.

4. InterStudy, *National HMO Census December 30, 1984* (Excelsior, Minn: Author, 1985), p. 5.

5. Penny L. Havlicek, *Medical Groups in the U.S., 1984* (Chicago: AMA Department of Survey Design and Analysis), 1985.

6. L.J. Freshnock and L.E. Jensen, "The Changing Pattern of Medical Group Practices in the United States 1969 to 1980" *Journal of the American Medical Association* 245, no. 21 (June 5, 1981): 2173–2176.

7. Leland R. Kaiser, "The Industry/Medical Group Interface," in *Meeting the Health Care Needs of Business: A Guide for Medical Groups,* ed. Bettina D. Kurowski (Denver: Center for Research in Ambulatory Health Care Administration), 1984.
8. Jon B. Christianson, Jan Malcolm, and Paul N. Ellwood, Jr., "The St. Louis Park Medical Center," *Medical Group Management* 26, no. 6 (November/December 1979).
9. J.H. Lorant and L.J. Kimball, "Determinants of Output in Group and Solo Medical Practice," *Health Services Research* 11 (Spring 1976): 6–20.
10. Center for Research in Ambulatory Health Care Administration, *The Group Practice Administrator Now and in the Future* (Denver: Author), 1979.
11. Mary Ziebell Soulier and Don T. DeCoster, "Productivity versus Cost Control: Considerations for Health Care Managers," *Health Care Management Review* (Winter 1982): 15–20.
12. *The Cost and Production Survey Report* (Denver: Medical Group Management Association), 1983, 1984, 1985.
13. *Physician Current Procedural Terminology,* 4th edition (Chicago: American Medical Association, updated annually).
14. Paul M. Ellwood, Jan K. Malcolm, and JoElyn McDonald, "Competition: Medicine's Creeping Revolution." Paper presented at the Sixth Private Sector Conference, Duke University Medical School, March 23, 1981 (Excelsior, Minn.: InterStudy), 1981.

REFERENCES

Ad Hoc Committee on the Cost of Medical Care, American Group Practice Association. "How Group Practice Can Help Hold Down Health Care Costs." *Group Practice* 28, no. 1 (January-February 1979): 12, 13, 31, 32.

American Group Practice Association, American Medical Association, and Medical Group Management Association. *Group Practice: Guidelines to Forming or Joining a Medical Group.* Denver: Center for Research in Ambulatory Health Care Administration, 1978.

Anderson, Gerard F. "Project Hope 'Data Watch.'" *Health Affairs* 4, no. 3 (Fall 1985): 100–107.

Arnett, Ross H. et al. "Health Spending Trends in the 1980s: Adjusting to Financial Incentives," *Health Care Financing Review* 6, no. 3 (Spring 1985).

Bendix, Jeff. "Ambulatory Care Centers Take Up Downtown Market." *Modern Healthcare* 12, no. 5 (May 1982): 17–18.

———. "Employers Prefer Negotiating Fees." *Modern Healthcare* 12, no. 5 (May 1982): 19–20.

Brudevold, Christine and David Plotnick. *A Survey of HMOs 1985.* Washington: Group Health Association of America, Inc., 1985.

Center for Research in Ambulatory Health Care Administration. *The Organization and Development of a Medical Group Practice.* Denver: Author, 1976.

"Concerns of Business Voiced to MDs." *American Medical News* 25, no. 6 (February 12, 1982): 3.

Cunningham, Lawrence F., and Katherine Blake. "Strategic Market Planning for Medical Group Practices," in *Meeting the Health Care Needs of Business: A Guide for Medical Groups,* edited by Bettina D. Kurowski. Denver: Center for Research in Ambulatory Health Care Administration, 1984.

———. "The Cost of Health Care: A Business Perspective," in *Meeting the Health Care Needs of Business: A Guide for Medical Groups,* edited by Bettina D. Kurowski. Denver: Center for Research in Ambulatory Health Care Administration, 1984.

Egdahl, Richard H. "Sounding Boards: Physicians and the Containment of Health-Care Costs." *New England Journal of Medicine* 304, no. 15 (April 9, 1981): 900–901.

Enthoven, Alain C. "Shattuck Lecture—Cutting Cost without Cutting the Quality of Care." *New England Journal of Medicine* 298, no. 22 (June 1, 1978): 1229–38.

Freeland, Mark S. and Carol E. Schendler. "Health Spending in the 1980s: Integration of Clinical Practice Patterns with Management," *Health Care Financing Review* 5, no. 3 (Spring 1984).

Harris, John M., Jr. *Role of the Medical Director in the Fee-for-Service/Prepaid Medical Group.* Going Prepaid Monograph Series. Denver: Center for Research in Ambulatory Health Care Administration, 1983.

Henderson, Cindy Walters, and Stephen J. Williams. *Medical Group Practice Assessment Manual.* Denver: Center for Research in Ambulatory Health Care Administration, 1979.

Kaiser, Leland R. *Take Charge of Your Destiny.* Denver: Center for Research in Ambulatory Health Care Administration, 1984. Videocassette.

Krill, Mary Alice and Barbara B. Gaugler. "Optimizing Your Effectiveness with the Board." *Medical Group Management* 30, no. 5 (September/October 1983): 10, 12, 14, 21.

Kropf, Roger. "Evaluating the Impact of Ambulatory Care on Health Care Costs." *Health Care Planning and Marketing* 1, no. 4 (January 1982): 25–38.

Levit, Katherine R. et al. "National Health Expenditures," *Health Care Financing Review* 7, no. 1 (Fall 1985).

McClain, Marion P. and E. Yvonne Spinson. "The Effects of Mode of Payment on the Use of Health Care Services among Patients Who Receive All or Part of Their Care under the Auspices of One Group of Physicians." Report of a study conducted by St. Louis Park Medical Center, 1980.

McNerney, Walter J. "Control of Health-Care Costs in the 1980s." *New England Journal of Medicine* 303, no. 19 (November 6, 1980): 1088–95.

Mechanic, David. "Approaches to Controlling the Costs of Medical Care: Short-Range and Long-Range Alternatives." *New England Journal of Medicine* 298, no. 5 (February 2, 1978): 249–54.

"Medicare, HMOs Jump 71 Percent; Enrollment Rises." *Hospitals,* March 20, 1986, p. 80.

Michaels, Joel L. *Legal Issues in the Fee-for-Service/Prepaid Medical Group.* Going Prepaid Monograph Series. Denver: Center for Research in Ambulatory Health Care Administration, 1984.

Naisbitt, John. *Megatrends.* New York: Warner Books, Inc., 1984.

NCHSR. "National Health Care Expenditure Study. Contacts with Physicians in Ambulatory Settings: Rates of Use, Expenditures, and Sources of Payment." *Data Preview* 16, U.S. Department of Health and Human Services Publication No. (PHS) 83-3361.

Neal, Patricia A. *Management Information Systems (MIS) in the Fee-for-Service/Prepaid Medical Group.* Going Prepaid Monograph Series. Denver: Center for Research in Ambulatory Health Care Administration, 1984.

Neumann, Bruce R. "Three Case Histories: A PPO, an HMO, and a Business/Health Coalition." In *Meeting the Health Care Needs of Business: A Guide for Medical Groups,* edited by Bettina D. Kurowski. Denver: Center for Research in Ambulatory Health Care Administration, 1984.

Nobrega, F.T., et al. "Development of Estimates of Utilization of Health Care Services in a Defined Population." Report to the Bureau of Health Planning of the Department of Health, Education, and Welfare. May 22, 1979. Contract Number (HRA) 231-77-0116.

Norris, Eileen. "Employers Use Various Remedies to Slash Surging Healthcare Costs." *Modern Healthcare* 11 (December 1981): 40, 42.

Olson, Donald R. *Impact of DRG Prospective Pricing on Medical Groups.* Denver: Center for Research in Ambulatory Health Care Administration, 1984. Videocassette.

Rorem, C. Rufus. *Private Group Clinics*. New York: Milbank Memorial Fund, 1971.

Rossiter, Louis, Alan Friedlob, and Kathryn Langwell. "Exploring Benefits of Risk-Based Contracting Under Medicare." *Healthcare Financial Management* 39, no. 5 (May 1985): 42–45, 48–50, 52, 54, 56, 58.

Schafer, Eldon L., Dwight J. Zulauf, and Michael E. Gocke. MBA, CPA. *Management Accounting for Fee-for-Service/Prepaid Medical Groups*. Denver: Center for Research in Ambulatory Health Care Administration, 1984.

Schafer, Eldon L., and Michael E. Gocke. *Management Accounting for Health Maintenance Organizations*. Denver: Center for Research in Ambulatory Health Care Administration, 1984.

Schafer, Eldon L., Dwight J. Zulauf, and Franklin L. McCarthy. *Practical Financial Management for Medical Groups*. Denver: Center for Research in Ambulatory Health Care Administration, 1979.

Shouldice, Robert G. *Marketing Management in the Fee-for-Service/Prepaid Medical Group*. Going Prepaid Monograph Series. Denver: Center for Research in Ambulatory Health Care Administration, 1984.

"The Spiraling Costs of Health Care: Rx: Competition." *Business Week* 2725 (February 8, 1982): 58–64.

Starr, Paul. *The Social Transformation of American Medicine*. New York: Basic Books, 1982.

Stevens, Edward B. *The History of the Medical Group Management Association*. Denver: Medical Group Management Association, 1976.

Suttun, H.L., Jr. and Allen J. Sorbo. *Actuarial Issues in the Fee-for-Service/Prepaid Medical Group*. Going Prepaid Monograph Series. Denver: Center for Research in Ambulatory Health Care Administration, 1984.

Tynan, Eileen A. "Provider Responses: Initiatives and Innovations." In *Meeting the Health Care Needs of Business: A Guide for Medical Groups*, edited by Bettina D. Kurowski. Denver: Center for Research in Ambulatory Health Care Administration, 1984, 17–24.

———. "Report of a Survey among Medical Groups on Alternative Health Systems for Business." In *Meeting the Health Care Needs of Business: A Guide for Medical Groups*, edited by Bettina D. Kurowski. Denver: Center for Research in Ambulatory Health Care Administration, 1984, 53–55.

U.S. General Accounting Office. *Report to the Secretary of Health and Human Services: Physician Cost-Containment Training Can Reduce Medical Costs*. February 4, 1982. Washington, DC: Government Printing Office, HRD 82-36.

Van Why, Robert H. *Preparing for Medicare Prospective Pricing of Physician Services*. Denver: Center for Research in Ambulatory Health Care Administration, 1984.

Chapter 7

A Nursing Administrative Perspective

Barbara J. Brown

If there is a single constant in today's complex health care services, it is the state of continuous change. The prospective payment system that became effective for hospital cost reporting years beginning on or after October 1, 1983 (P.L. 97-248, the Tax Equity and Fiscal Responsibility Act (TEFRA)) has changed nurses' lives considerably. These changes were absolutely necessary if health care costs, those incurred by both the federal government and by all other parties, were to be brought under control. Payment based on costs had to be eliminated. Even though the hospital industry had voluntary cost containment, promoted since 1979, there was no easy way in which marketplace incentives and penalties could stop the spiraling costs of health care.

The previous payment system of cost reimbursement actually had helped increase costs. It offered no incentive to operate less expensively when greater revenues could be obtained simply by increasing costs. As a result of the inflation of the medical care dollar, 50 percent to 60 percent of all Medicare expenditures since 1965 went to higher payments for providers (hospitals and doctors) rather than for any improvement in public benefits. Additional coverages were not made available for older persons.[1] The cause of this spiral was cost reimbursement and fee-for-service payment to physicians. It was essential, therefore, to shift the economic risk from third parties to providers. The result was the diagnosis related group (DRG) case-mix reimbursement system and the transfer of risk from the government to the hospitals.

On the negative side, the DRGs faced two problems: (1) the fear that some form of health care rationing will occur, and (2) access to care will be reduced because some hospitals will close while others may set quotas on the number of patients, especially the costly Medicare clients. Both factors have implications for malpractice in that providers can decide to limit much needed services, thereby denying a patient access or can determine not to provide service because of the client's lack of financial resources or lack of coverage by insurance, creating increased debt for the hospital. The question arises as to whether physicians and hospitals are the most appropriate rationers of health care. Next, if they are, what risks do they face? According to the report by the President's Commission for the Study of Ethical Problems in Medicine and Biomedical and Behavioral Research, "differences in the availability of health services (securing access to health care) was a responsibility of society."[2]

Prior to DRGs, caregivers had few economic constraints. Today, if health care providers must consider the purse strings, patients may lose trust in caregivers.

NURSING'S ROLE AND RESPONSIBILITIES

Nursing's responsibility in cost-efficient management is to identify its products and program outputs in relation to patient care. To do this, some programs such as obstetrics might be eliminated—some product lines that are not compatible with patient care priorities or simply are not affordable. Nurses are promoting products using sophisticated marketing techniques in development of increased patient volume and revenue. The concentration is on the bottom line—the net income for long-term financial survivability or liability. Benefits are limited and demand for acute care facilities is decreasing because decisions are being made to give up some programs. Home care, extended care, day care, short stay services, and other less costly delivery services are increasing. The need to focus resources where they count requires that nursing management participate in analysis of the institution's strengths and weaknesses, identify the principle issues, and establish priorities.

To integrate clinical and financial data, attention should be focused on nursing, the number of nurses, and the skills required. This attention will lead management to develop more computerized nursing systems. The information generated will determine earlier patient placement in accommodation beds or home health programs to replace acute hospital utilization. To do this, sound financially and clinically integrated nursing data are essential.

The data are not necessarily factors represented by DRGs. They involve planning, managing, and communication with all providers and responding to the constant changes. It is necessary to analyze nursing's efforts as they relate to a specific patient on a particular day, to specific procedures, and to nursing care needs. The quality of the data—their dependability, understandability, availability, flexibility of analysis, timeliness, and cost—are essential when dealing with clinical-financial data base information.

Unfortunately, nursing generally is a lesser priority in information systems than are other clinical data streams. Therefore, time is a major consideration in fully integrating nursing into the clinical and financial data base. Nursing administrators cannot wait to begin collecting the data and implementing a system because it takes two years or more just to develop quality analysis.

Walker's studies on the cost of nursing care in hospitals postulate two questions: (1) How should the relative cost of nursing care be determined? (2) Are all expenditures in the nursing services' operating budgets specifically related to direct or indirect nursing care services?[3] He sorts out comparative costs of nursing care versus nonnursing care and breaks down daily room rates and hospital services. He reports that nursing care accounted for only about half of the daily room charge for intensive care units (ICUs) and may be significantly less in other areas of the hospital. For the six diagnostic categories examined in the study, nursing accounted for 20 percent or less of total hospital charges. This is quite different from the common belief that the cost of nursing care is almost synonymous with daily room charges. The question of how to determine nursing costs will remain without a definitive answer until unsound fiscal practices such as placing nursing care costs and revenues with room and board are abandoned.[4] More extensive studies of nursing costs must be done.

Sovie et al. report that nursing needs of the individual patients within the DRGs are extremely variable, as reflected by the large standard deviations in average nursing hours associated with the DRGs.[5] The broad range is indicated by the minimum and maximum nursing hours and the high coefficient variance for these average nursing hours.[6]

DRGs AND THEIR PROBLEMS

DRGs, while found to constitute a useful classification for both nursing research and management, are not accurate measures of nursing resource consumption. It is well recognized that the assistance of information systems technology is needed to develop and track DRGs or product data and costs. As noted, the need for the automation and integration of nursing into financial and clinical data systems cannot be overemphasized. However, as the study by Sovie et al. points out, the lack of homogeneity of nursing acuity within the DRGs, as reflected by the large standard deviations of the average nursing hours and the broad range of hours descriptive of patients' nursing needs within DRGs, warrants further prompt study.[7]

What is the effect of length of stay on this heterogeneity of nursing care hours within DRGs? It is necessary to consider the efficacy of nursing practice associated with specific DRGs just as much as the efficacy of medical care. Computerized information systems will uncover the basic elements but the key to success is a valid and reliable patient classification system.

Patient classification may be defined as a grouping of patients according to some observable or inferred properties or characteristics. It is a method of categorizing or grouping a particular population into various levels based on predetermined or predefined factors, variables, or patient conditions. The traditional and primary purpose of a classification system is to categorize patients into various levels of need, care, or medical status so the nursing department can allocate, monitor, justify, and assess proper staffing distribution.

There are, obviously, any number of possibilities for types of classification. For example:

- Medical classification systems use such characteristics as blood type, medical specialty, diagnoses, and insurance coverage to categorize patients, with each classification serving some unique function.
- Patient classification in nursing means categorization according to assessment of patients' nursing care requirements over a specified time, with the purpose of assigning nursing personnel.

To encompass both the definition and the purpose, the term "patient classification system" is commonly used. The development of such systems has been in response to the enormous number and types of patient care demands nurses must respond to. There may be wide swings in need for specific interventions from day to day and from shift to shift, fluctuations that are independent of the number of patients in the unit or their medical diagnoses. Because the number of patients in a unit may not be an adequate indicator of the demand for care, grouping them into categories that reflect the consumption of service time provides a more rational and sensitive approach to determining the care requirements.

Joint Commission on the Accreditation of Hospitals (JCAH) Standard 3 states:[8]

> The Nursing Department assignments in the provision of nursing care shall be commensurate with the qualifications of nursing personnel and shall be designed to meet the nursing care needs of patients.

The Interpretation of the JCAH Accreditation Manual for 1985 states:[9]

> The Nursing Department shall define, implement and maintain a system for determining patient requirements for patient care on the basis of demonstrated patient need, appropriate nursing intervention and priority of care. Specific nursing personnel staffing for each nursing care unit, including, as appropriate, surgical suite, obstetrical suite, ambulatory care department, and emergency department shall be commensurate with the patient care requirement, staff expertise, unit geography, availability of support services and method of patient care delivery. The hospital admission system should allow for input from the Nursing Department in coordinating patient requirements for nursing care with available nursing resources.

The primary use is to make staffing decisions from an allocation standpoint; that is, deciding which units will receive extra staff or which ones will not have the full complement scheduled initially. Once the nurses are on the unit, patient classification, which is translated to hours of care, is used to make patient assignments for each nurse based on acuity, providing a more even work distribution per nurse.

The information obtained from data analysis can be used in a variety of ways. For example:

- long-range budgeting for staffing needs
- developing staffing for projected units
- tracking trends in patient population and staffing
- tracking individual patient acuity
- determining how the patient dollar is spent in relation to nursing care
- billing separately for nursing services based on level of care required (patient care classification)
- relating nursing costs to DRGs
- determining what other types of patient care units need to be developed, such as cooperative care units, hospice, short-term rehabilitation care, etc.
- correlating patient diagnoses with patient classification levels.

PATIENT CLASSIFICATION: 2 SYSTEMS

Two types of patient classifications are in use: the Prototype System and the Factor Evaluation System. The Prototype System generally is considered to be the more subjective of the two. It uses broad descriptions, generally has three to five exclusive levels, and workload is predetermined for each level. It is simple, and certain key descriptors place a patient in a specific category of care. For example, a patient on a cardiac monitor, regardless of condition—from very acute to impending discharge—would be considered a Category 3 in a prototype evaluation system simply because of the cardiac monitor. That one indicator automatically assigns the patient to a predetermined category. The estimated patient care time for each category also is predetermined. The advantages of a Prototype System are that it is easy to use, costs less to develop, and is good for homogeneous populations. The disadvantages are that if a unit has a heterogeneous population, the system is not specific enough to be useful and it is very difficult to test the validity and reliability of the system.

The second major type, the Factor Evaluation System, uses specific characteristics or attributes that define the classification level through a process of summing or checking off each of the particular characteristics. A determination of projected patient care is then arrived at by translating the score to hours of care.

The major difference is that rather than the category's being defined, each individual factor has a weighting that is related somehow to a measure of care time. Each patient is rated individually and there are any number of ratings that could be arrived upon—for example from 1 to 150—that would describe the level of care needed for that person. The advantages of this type of system are that it contains more finite data and more sophistication, which makes possible the interpretation for some of the more complex analyses, such as cost accounting. It is less subjective, since a patient's category is based on the combination of individual factors rather than on the predetermined definition of this person as a Class 3. Disadvantages of the system are that it is costly to develop and must be tailored to the individual institution, with time studies, etc., in order to be valid and reliable. The individual nurse caring for the patient also must take a few minutes of time to classify patients properly.

The factors or critical indicators used to describe nursing care requirements have different meanings for nursing practice and process. Critical is not used in the medical sense; instead, it refers to the components that are most crucial for correct identification of the appropriate category of nursing care. Since the primary purpose of patient classification is to determine the need for nursing care resources, the critical indicators represent activities that have the greatest impact on nursing care time. Other activities can be projected to occur during the shift, as against the possible unexpected time-consuming activities.

Observational studies of nursing care have helped identify these critical indicators. Typically, they include nursing activities associated with feeding, bathing, and ambulation. Others include those involving preoperative preparation, observation, special treatments, and incontinence care. Indicators also focus on mental as well as physical well-being, teaching interventions, care planning, and discharge planning for home care as well as family support.

THE VIRGINIA MASON SYSTEM

Virginia Mason Hospital in Seattle has had a patient classification system since 1970, since then refining it to include specialty units such as the ICU, the CCU, the Rehabilitation Unit and the Oncology Unit (see Appendix 7–A).

In 1974 the Patient Classification and Nursing Utilization System (PCNU) was introduced. It was designed to predict staffing requirements per unit per shift by categorizing patients into one of four weighted categories. Information on predicted staff levels and providing staff was then entered into the hospital computer to provide a monthly nursing utilization report. A basic management engineering work sampling technique was used to develop this system. When the specialized patient classification systems were developed, it became clear that the PCNU was not meeting the needs but it nonetheless was continued. Tracking data did show increased acuity even though staffing according to these indicators was less reliable.

Tracking patients over time demonstrates that the medical-surgical acuity scores for the more acute patients have been increasing steadily (see Figure 7–1). For example, in 1974 those in Class 1, the less acute group, comprised 28 percent of the patient population; by 1985, Class 1 patients were less than 2 percent of the population. Class 2 patients, who in 1974 were 37 percent of the population, decreased to 25 percent. However, Class 3 patients, who in 1974 were 27 percent of the population, had increased to 53 percent by 1985. Class 4 patients, the most acute, went from 7 percent in 1974 to 20 percent in 1985. The data indicate that patients in the more acute categories are sicker, take more time, and consume more resources than in 1974.

In 1980, Virginia Mason Hospital used the specifics of patient acuity and oncology to justify to the Washington State Hospital Commission a need for more full-time equivalents to deliver quality cancer care to patients. With the increased complexity of care problems, and with improved technology and methodology for analyzing and predicting the use of staff for patients, it is important that patient classification systems be recognized as containing significant data for hospitals' presentations to rate-setting commissions as well as in analyzing DRGs.

To illustrate the difficulty in establishing nursing care requirements for any given diagnosis, the following three cases are presented with the oncology patient

Figure 7–1 Daily Averages, Percentage of Total Number of Patients

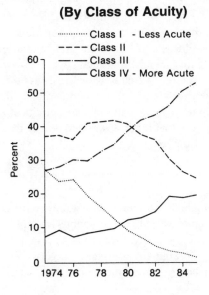

(By Class of Acuity)

classification system. Each of these patients had acute leukemia, but their needs for nursing support services varied considerably.

Patient A

This 67-year-old female, who had been a registered nurse, was admitted on August 31, 1985, with the diagnosis of acute myelogenous leukemia. She was scheduled to receive two weeks of continuous infusion of a single chemotherapeutic agent (ARA-C). She had never had chemotherapy, nor had she spent longer than two weeks in a hospital. She had been told to expect a total hospitalization of about a month.

Because of myriad unexpected and unpredictable complications, her total hospital stay extended more than ten weeks. The chemotherapy did not control her leukemia, she developed a number of infections that required multiple antibiotics, and, as with all similar patients, she received multiple red blood cell and platelet transfusions. She developed adverse reactions on several occasions to the platelet transfusions that required intravenous medication for control. Other manifestations of her illness and treatment included painful lesions in the mouth, pain at the site of multiple bone marrow aspirations, severe headaches, and pronounced fatigue and nausea that interfered with daily living activities, including eating and ambulation.

When it became apparent that the chemotherapy was not controlling her leukemia, she was told that her prognosis was not hopeful and that she had limited time left in her life. She began to process her grief by recounting significant events in her life. She shared her feelings with nursing staff about dying and leaving her family and friends. However, she felt it important to remain cheerful when her family was present, so that much of the sharing was done with the nurses. The patient's needs to express these concerns could not be ignored; at the same time, her husband and other family members needed support. It seemed too painful for the family members to share their concerns or to discuss the problem openly.

Because of her prolonged hospitalization and bed rest, she needed assistance and encouragement with food intake and self-care activities. Despite her career as a R.N., her illness interfered with her desire and ability to care for herself, thus increasing her use of nursing resources.

Patient B

This 19-year-old college sophomore was admitted in September 1985 for treatment of a newly diagnosed acute myelogenous leukemia. She had just started the fall semester at a local university. Her parents accompanied her, offering her support in the hospital's foreign environment. Surgery was necessary for placement of a right atrial catheter, a small tube that allows central venous access for treatment and transfusions. She received several intravenous and oral anti-neoplastic drugs in a specific sequence over a two-week period. The nursing staff taught her about the side effects of the medications and prepared her for what to expect. These side effects included loss of hair, anemia, lowered defense to infection, an increased tendency to bleed, fatigue, mouth sores, nausea, vomiting, loss of appetite, tingling and numbness of her extremities, diarrhea, etc.

She required blood product support over her one-month hospitalization but developed reactions to the platelet transfusions that required intravenous medication for control. She also developed a systemic yeast infection that was treated with a potent intravenous medication, and to this, too, she had an adverse reaction. She experienced a nagging headache for an extended time. Monitoring her vital signs as well as her comfort and safety during all of these reactions was an integral role of the nursing staff.

Her parents were an important source of support for this patient. However, they were concerned with her changing status and her struggle to get well. They asked many questions and expressed their feelings to medical and nursing staff. The patient herself was quite concerned with the loss of hair, loss of time from school, and distance from friends. Part of nursing care was to listen and offer support and encouragement to both the patient and her parents.

Patient C

This young woman in her early 20s was admitted in October 1985 for treatment of newly diagnosed acute leukemia. After surgical placement of an intravenous catheter, she received similar oral and intravenous antineoplastic agents over a two-week period. As with other patients, nursing instructed her and counseled her regarding expectations from treatment and potential side effects.

This patient had never experienced a serious, life-threatening illness but faced this with great inner strength and determination to not be ill. She eagerly partici-pated in her care and experienced minimal side effects from her chemotherapeutic program. She had great support from her large family, whose members appeared to face her illness as she did—with an attitude that one had to get through.

Not until three and a half weeks into her treatment did she show signs of infection. She did not have adverse reactions to the multiple blood products she received, and she chose not to disguise the loss of her hair. She maintained her ability and interest in eating, and performing regular exercises. She handled the tediousness of hospital life with resourcefulness, and her self-sufficiency clearly decreased her nursing care needs.

PREDICTIVE STAFFING REQUIREMENTS

These three cases demonstrated that nursing care requirements cannot be determined on the basis of a single medical diagnosis; each shared the same medical problem but consumed greatly different degrees of nursing support (see Figure 7–2). The Oncology Patient Classification System based on Roy's adaptation model[10] clearly provides for predictive staffing requirements as well as sensitivity in responding to special needs and demands of the terminally ill. Roy's adaptation model views humans as biopsychosocial beings who function as a totality and are in constant interaction with a continually changing internal and external environment.

Roy describes individuals as constituting open adaptive systems in which their environment provides the stimuli to those open systems. Thus, adaptation, both as process and end state, is a response to the environment that promotes individuals' general goals. Five human components are identified within this model: biological, psychological, cultural, social, and spiritual.

The incorporation of the Roy adaptation model as the foundation of the oncological patient classification system led to the effective addressing of patient care needs specific to that population in order to determine nursing care requirements (patient acuity). The model is redefined into seven components, specifically for the purposes of patient classification: physiological, psychological, sociocultural, spiritual, patient-teaching, discharge planning, and patient care evaluation and satisfaction. This focuses the design of the system around the patient. It also serves as a model for assessment by specifically defining various factors under each component that are specific to the oncological nursing care unit's needs. This approach makes possible the incorporation of oncological nursing philosophy, goals, objectives, and patient care planning in the patient classification system.

The oncological patient classification system (Exhibit 7–1) has proved to be a cost-effective management tool to relate budgetary controls to policies and procedures for oncology practice. It also is used as a guide for nursing care planning.

Figure 7–2 Acute Myelogenous Leukemia: Nursing Support Needs

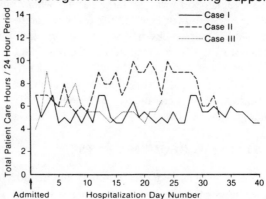

The system provides an effective means for monitoring productivity and appropriate allocation of staffing resources. It also has been used for variable billing.

On the Oncology Unit at Virginia Mason Medical Center, many patients are on cancer research protocols initiated by certain physicians. These protocols require increased nursing care. Therefore, individual physicians drive the cost of nursing upward while the reimbursement has remained limited. To compensate for the increased consumption of nursing resources, the implementation of a variable billing system based on a patient classification system in oncology was initiated in 1983. This has permitted additional staffing, with further reimbursement obtained for the increased level of care needed to provide these patients with optimal services.

The special oncology nursing care charge (Exhibit 7–2) is analogous to private duty nursing payment by patients in years past. At Virginia Mason, revenue generated from this source from September to December 1983 was $30,800, in 1984 $89,740, and in 1985 $116,731. These revenues exceeded the costs of increasing the staff needed to deliver the extra care predicted by the patient classification system.

VARIABLE BILLING

In addition, the development of a nursing impact statement (Exhibit 7–3) to estimate the cost in hours of care added by clinical research protocols afforded an information base to be considered in the manager's budget process. While the Virginia Mason Patient Classification System in Oncology is a form of variable billing, other such systems also have been used in similar billing.

Higgerson and Van Slyck report that the advantages of variable billing for nursing care include identifying revenue nursing cost centers and facilitating systematic control of revenue and expenses to improve budget planning and management. It also generates a tremendous amount of data that can be used in administrative planning and decision making. It is more equitable than past billing practices for the patient, the third party payer, and the hospital, making it a public relations asset.

However, in times of DRGs, the disadvantages of the system are that it makes no difference when there is a case mix or set payment, and charges at one hospital are not easily compared with those of another any more than they are with the DRG approach. The mix of patients with varying classification has a significant effect on revenue, thus increasing the possibility of lower income. "There is some question as to whether there is good accountability for nursing to actually deliver the care."[11]

Whenever nursing attempts to bill for its service, there must be integrity in the system; that is, if the patient is charged for a level of nursing care, it is imperative

Exhibit 7–1 Oncology Patient Classification System

M ONCOLOGY PATIENT CLASSIFICATION FORM
VIRGINIA MASON HOSPITAL

PATIENT NAME

Date _____
Report prepared by _____
Shift – Day for Evening ( ), Evening for Night ( ), Night for Day ( )

ROOM & PATIENT

	PATIENT CARE NEEDS	Weights	58	59	60	62	63¹	63²	64	65¹	65²	66	67	68	69	73¹	73²
CHEMOTHERAPY (Choose one)	1 Most Complicated	5															
	2 Moderately Complicated	3															
	3 Least Complicated	1															
PAIN MANAGEMENT (Choose one)	4 Occasional	1															
	5 Stable	2															
	6 Unstable	5															
IV AND MED ADMINISTRATION	7 Difficult PO/via tube/Insulin	# X1															
	8 IV Partial Fills	# X2															
	9 IV Blood	# X5															
	10 PRN MED/N & V/Sedation	# X2															
	11 IV/HA/CVP	# X2															
TUBE MANAGEMENT	12 Foley	2															
	13 N/G	3															
	14 Chest Tube	4															
	15 Hickman line (non self-care)	4															
	16 IBI	4															
	17 Insertion of Tube by RN	# X2															
NURSING ASSESSMENT	18 Vital Signs (T,P,R, BP)	# X1															
	19 Intake and Output	# X2															
	20 Weights (bed scale only)	2															
	21 Urine/Stool/Sputum Testing	# X1															
AMBULATION OF PATIENT	22 Ambulation with Assistance	# X2															
	23 BRP/Commode with Assistance	# X2															
	24 Bedrest (turn/ROM/Bedpan)	# X3															
BOWEL AND BLADDER PROGRAM	25 Bowel Program	4															
	26 Bladder Program	# X3															
	27 Ostomy Care	# X5															
NUTRITION	28 Tube Feeding	# X1															
	29 Total Feeding by Staff (DX2, EX1)	3															
HYGIENE	30 Complete Bedbath	4															
	31 Assisted Shower	2															
	32 Special Oral Care	# X1															
REPIRATORY CARE	33 Suction via N/T/Trac.	# X3															
	34 Suction Nasally	# X2															
	35 Bennett Treatment	# X1															
	36 Resperex Treatment	# X1															
	37 Oxygen Mask/Prongs	# X1															
CARE PRECAUTIONS	38 Wound and Dressing Care	# X2															
	39 Isolation	3															
MENTAL STATUS	40 Confused/Combative	1															
	41 Restraints and Observe	3															
	42 Continual Observation	6															
PSYCHOSOCIAL ASSESSMENT	43 Assessment and Evaluation	# X2															
	44 Activities	3															
	45 Referrals	# X2															
DISCHARGE PLANNING	46 Assessment of goals, obj. & planning	# X3															
	47 Meeting with Patient/Family	4															
	48 Phone calls/referrals/follow-up	# X2															
TEACHING NEEDS	49 Assessment and Planning	# X2															
	50 Teaching	# X3															
	51 Evaluation	# X2															
SPIRITUAL NEED	52 Spiritual comfort for patient/family	# X2															
SOCIO-CULTURAL NEEDS	53 Special Food Requirement	1															
	54 Communication Barrier	2															
	55 Unit Constant	3	3	3	3	3	3	3	3	3	3	3	3	3	3	3	3
	56 Identified 1:1 (one to one)	✓															
	57 Admission/transfer to unit	✓															
	58 Discharge/transfer from unit	✓															
	59 ACUITY SCORE																
	60 ACUITY CLASSIFICATION																
	61 PATIENT CARE HOURS																

74	75^1	75^2	76	77^1	77^2	78	79^1	79^2	80	82		
3	3	3	3	3	3	3	3	3	3	3	3	3

Calculation Area

I ___ ≶PCH ÷ 8 = _______ Patient Care Providers

II Pending Admits Chemo _____ other _____
Pending Discharges _____

III

SCHEDULED STAFF

Days			Evenings			Nights		
NCC	RN	LPN	NCC	RN	LPN	NCC	RN	LPN
Plus		– W.S. – N.A.	Plus		– W.S. – N.A.	Plus		– W.S. – N.A.

IV

	ACUITY CLASS					Total Number of Patients
	I	II	III	IV	V	
Number of Patients:						

V Do you feel that the **predicted** staffing for the **oncoming** shift is adequate? Y _____ N _____
If not, what changes would you have made?

Comments:

VI Did you feel that the number of nurses provided on **your** shift was adequate? Y _____ N _____
If not, what changes would you have made?

Comments:

CONVERSION TABLE

Acuity Class	I	II	III	IV	V
Acuity Score	≤ 24	25-35	36-45	46-59	≥ 60
Patient Care Hours	1.5	2	3	4	6

FM-427 Rev. 5-83

Exhibit 7–2 Oncology Special Care Charge

Definition:	An Oncology Special Care condition applies to any patient on 8-East requiring four or more patient care hours per shift for one or more shifts. Leukemia patients, bone marrow transplant patients, and terminal patients can consistently require four or more patient care hours per shift. Patients receiving intensive antineoplastic chemotherapy, frequent intravenous medications (antiemetics or antibiotics), or blood have a high potential for needing four or more patient care hours per shift.
	Patient care hours include direct and indirect care. The hours are identified through use of the Virginia Mason Hospital Oncology Classification Form (see Exhibit 7–1).
Assumptions:	1. Any bed on 8-East can be used for activating the Oncology Special Care Charge.
	2. The activation of the Oncology Special Care Charge is a clinical decision initiated by Nursing with subsequent agreement by Medicine.
	3. The number of Oncology Special Care patients on 8-East will vary from shift to shift. There will be no minimum or maximum number.
	4. The ability to activate the special charge requires a commitment to deliver additional nursing hours.
	5. The Oncology Special Care Charge will be assigned to patients on 8-East only.
	6. The minimum period of time for the Special Care Charge will be four hours.
	7. The assessment of even twenty-four hours of the Oncology Special Care Charge incurs less expense for patients than if patients were transferred to the Intensive Care Unit.
Guidelines for Use:	1. Beginning September 8, 1983, all patients on 8-East requiring four or more patient care hours per shift will be assigned the Oncology Special Care Charge.
	2. The physician is responsible for noting this status on the physician's order sheet in the medical record. The need for this status will also be documented in the progress record.
	3. The evening ward secretary is responsible for preparing a daily summary of Oncology Special Care Charge patients (based on the Oncology Patient Classification Form) and forwarding it to Revenue.
	4. If a patient who has been assigned an Oncology Special Care Charge dies, the evening ward secretary will note the time of death on the appropriate daily summary.
	5. As established by the Finance Department, a $10.00/hour charge is assigned to all patients on 8-East requiring four or more patient care hours per shift.

Exhibit 7–3 Nursing Impact Statement

(Inpatient Studies Only)

A. Nursing Facilities
  1. Which nursing units will be utilized? _____
  2. Which shifts will be involved? _____
  3. What will be the site of data collection (for example, patient bedside, special procedure area)?_____
  _____
  4. What equipment will be used during the study that would involve nursing monitoring?
  _____

B. Present Clinical Practices
  1. What are the proposed dates of data collection? _____
  2. What tasks would the nurses be performing within this protocol?
  _____
  3. What will be the nursing time to be utilized per each day of data collection:
  Nursing time required per 24 hours: _____hours _____minutes
  4. Does this research project budget include nursing time cost?
  Yes_____ No_____ If no, what sources will be funding the nursing time utilized in the study? _____
  _____
  5. Who is responsible on the research project team to explain the study, instruct staff, etc., to the nursing staff?
  Name _____
  Title _____Phone _____

C. Future Clinical Practice
  1. What are the implications in the study that would affect patient care and/or nursing care in the future (if applicable)? _____
  _____
  2. What additional information would assist in evaluating nursing impact? _____
  _____

Please contact Ann Reiner, extension 4208, for any questions regarding the nursing impact statement.
Nursing impact statement approved _____
Cochairperson of Nursing Research Committee _____
Clinical director _____Unit _____

that nurses actually deliver that level of care and that patient and family members can validate that they received the sufficient amount of care billed. There is little that is questionable in intensive and critical care units, but in general medical-surgical units these variables must be defined more clearly than the workload index models have allowed for.

Further development at Virginia Mason Hospital in patient classification resulted in a redirection in the medical-surgical classification system based on the

Carnevali Planning Model. That model describes nursing as a discipline concerned with two major groups of phenomena and the relationship between them.[12] The major categories of central concern are daily living and functional health status.[13] In developing the medical/surgical patient classification instrument (Exhibit 7–4) for Virginia Mason, ten other hospitals from rural Washington participated as members of the Health Services Consortium, which is based at Virginia Mason Medical Center. (Forms for additional systems are presented in Appendix 7–A.)

Staff nurses in all participating hospitals developed critical indicators in the areas of living in transition, activities of daily living, daily living with symptom management, biomedical requirements (signs and indicators, including IV and medication administration, tube management, respiratory care, surgical care, and bowel and bladder program), and health promotion and maintenance. Critical indicators in health promotion and maintenance include teaching needs, psychosocial support, life style modification, and discharge planning/home care, which often is overlooked.

This instrument was tested in hospitals of 30, 60, and 100 beds, and a 336-bed tertiary care institution. It had the potential to lead to a significant breakthrough in information systems in nursing. When the same instrument can be used to create data sets to analyze consumption of nursing resources in a variety of patient care settings, it will be a beginning of a common data base in patient classification systems. This data base will allow for comparisons for planning and forecasting budgets and their submission to hospital rate commissions. In addition, it will allow for costing out of nursing and comparing resource consumption by DRG number. The specifics of nursing resource consumption add to the overall fiduciary responsibilities of nurse executives. This includes preparation, monitoring, and controlling the budget.

THE ROLE OF THE BUDGET

The budget is a tool for allocating resources and communicating predictions of the future. It also measures actual activity against stated objectives.

Because the Medicare prospective payment system uses an average per day nursing cost, the next significant work in reimbursement will be centered on breaking out nursing costs and creating variable billing systems in that area. This, coupled with a quality medical record data base that is accessible, dependable, and timely, will help in the development of standards by which to evaluate the data and their accumulation. A national data stream for nursing care delivery would be highly desirable.

Data streams for nursing are being identified. In a 1985 conference on Minimum Data Sets for Nursing sponsored by the University of Wisconsin-Milwaukee, elements were developed comparable with those already being collected, such as uniform hospital discharge data. The data included nursing diagnosis, intervention, outcome, and intensity of care. The patient or client demographic data included personal identification, date of birth, sex, race and ethnicity, and residence. The service data included the unique numbers of the facility or service agency, patient or client, and principal registered nurse provider, plus the episode admission or encounter date, discharge or termination date, disposition of patient or client, and expected payer for most of the bill.[14]

The key issue is to classify patients into disease categories to ensure equity in the charging reimbursement process. Various patients consume nursing resource categories that may not correlate with disease categories. Such data are essential in the DRG reimbursement procedures. Nursing care is predicated on both the medical diagnosis and the nursing diagnosis. However, the important factor is that patients with similar medical problems receive comparable treatment that is comparably charged. The initial presumption in DRGs is that the care given to those individuals for whom more resources are used has been either unnecessary or less sufficiently given, creating an "outlier."

What kind of administrative involvement can take place in the integration of financial, managerial, and clinical information system? A new emphasis or justification for strategic planning takes on a different priority in 1986. Important aspects of planning and financial analysis include the consideration of new and expensive technologies. There has been much improvement in health care technologies since the mid-1970s and that will continue to the end of the century but will be slower because of restricted funding. The rapid advances in the use of computers and electronics to help solve medical problems will require efficiency and cost effectiveness before third party payers and the public will pay for them. This becomes a major moral issue in applying cost/benefit analysis to medical technology. Any technology that develops noninvasive procedures or diagnoses and treatment, such as the Extracorporeal Shockwave Lithotripter, will be well rewarded.

The lithotripter team is multidisciplinary, consisting of managers, technicians, nurses, doctors, and financial experts. It is in the position to make the right decisions regarding this new technology. Data are analyzed in relation to the resources deployed in order to understand the dynamics of the health care system and control the cost in relationship to such issues as relative benefits, risks, and access.

Administrators also find that the medical record is an adequate clinical document that serves as input to the medical management information system. It also must be entered in the nursing management system. Nurses are in position to make the process concurrent rather than historical. They have a major role in utilization control and must establish their importance in case-mix control. They need a broadened education in finances, information systems, and general management.

Exhibit 7–4 Medical/Surgical Patient Classification System

MEDICAL / SURGICAL
PATIENT CLASSIFICATION
VIRGINIA MASON HOSPITAL

DATE _____
UNIT _____

☐ NIGHTS FOR DAYS
☐ DAYS FOR EVENINGS
☐ EVENINGS FOR NIGHTS

Multiply X1 for Minimum Assist
Multiply X2 for Moderate Assist
Multiply X3 for Maximum Assist
Patient Name
Room

Category		Critical Indicators	Scale	Weight						
LIVING IN TRANSITION		1 Admission / History and Assessment		4						
		2 Discharge		2						
		3 Transfer		2						
		4 Indirect Care / Care Planning		5	5	5	5	5	5	5
ACTIVITIES OF DAILY LIVING		5 Nutrition	X	2 X#						
		6 Hygiene	X	2						
		7 Mobility	X	2						
		8 Communication	X	1						
DAILY LIVING WITH SYMPTOM MANAGEMENT		9 Sensory Deficit	X	1						
		10 Alteration in Level of Consciousness	X	1						
		11 Safety Precautions	X	1						
		12 Anxiety/Agitation/Depression	X	1						
		13 Nausea / Vomiting	X	1						
		14 Alteration in Respiratory Status	X	1						
		15 Pain	X	1						
		16 Isolation	X	1						
B I O M E D I C A L R E Q U I R E M E N T S	SIGNS AND INDICATORS	17 Vital Signs/Assessment		1 X#						
		18 Postural BPs		1 X#						
		19 Intake and Output		1 X#						
		20 Weights		1						
		21 Blood / Urine / Stool / Sputum Testing		1 X#						
		22 Cardiac Monitor		2						
		23 Neuro Check		1 X#						
	IV AND MEDICATION ADMINISTRATION	24 PRN Medication/Insulin		1 X#						
		25 Complicated Medications		2 X#						
		26 Partial Fills / Intermittent IV Meds		1 X#						
		27 Hickman/Chemo/CVP		3 X#						
		28 Start IV		2						
		29 Continuous IVs / Hep Loc		1 X#						
		30 Blood Draw (Central Line)		1						
		31 Monitored IV Drugs / Blood Administration		2 X#						
	TUBE MANAGEMENT	32 Gravity Drainage Tube		1 X#						
		33 Suction Drainage Tube		1 X#						
		34 Tube Irrigation		1 X#						
		35 Insertion of Tube/Procedure Assist		3 X#						
	RESPIRATORY CARE	36 Suction via NT / Trach.		1 X#						
		37 Tracheostomy Care		2 X#						
		38 Respiratory Treatment		1 X#						
	SURGICAL CARE	39 Pre-Op Care		3						
		40 Post-Op Care	X	1						
		41 Wound and Dressing Care	X	1 X#						
	BOWEL AND BLADDER PROGRAM	42 Bowel Program	X	1						
		43 Bladder Care	X	1						
		44 Ostomy Care	X	1						
HEALTH PROMOTION AND MAINTENANCE		45 Teaching Needs	X	2						
		46 Psycho-Social Support	X	1						
		47 Lifestyle Modification	X	1						
		48 Discharge Planning / Home Care	X	2						
ACUITY SCORE										
PATIENT CARE HOURS										

FM 28 Rev 8/85

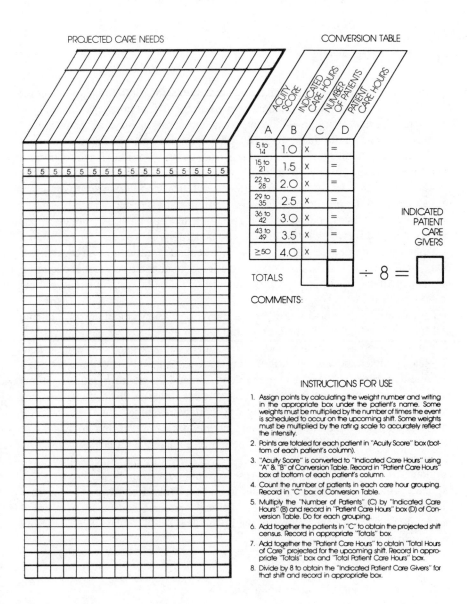

PROJECTED CARE NEEDS

CONVERSION TABLE

	A	B	C	D
ACUITY SCORE / INDICATED CARE HOURS / NUMBER OF PATIENTS / PATIENT CARE HOURS				
5 to 14	1.0	x		=
15 to 21	1.5	x		=
22 to 28	2.0	x		=
29 to 35	2.5	x		=
36 to 42	3.0	x		=
43 to 49	3.5	x		=
≥50	4.0	x		=
TOTALS				

÷ 8 = □

INDICATED PATIENT CARE GIVERS

COMMENTS:

INSTRUCTIONS FOR USE

1. Assign points by calculating the weight number and writing in the appropriate box under the patient's name. Some weights must be multiplied by the number of times the event is scheduled to occur on the upcoming shift. Some weights must be multiplied by the rating scale to accurately reflect the intensity.

2. Points are totaled for each patient in "Acuity Score" box (bottom of each patient's column).

3. "Acuity Score" is converted to "Indicated Care Hours" using "A" & "B" of Conversion Table. Record in "Patient Care Hours" box at bottom of each patient's column.

4. Count the number of patients in each care hour grouping. Record in "C" box of Conversion Table.

5. Multiply the "Number of Patients" (C) by "Indicated Care Hours" (B) and record in "Patient Care Hours" box (D) of Conversion Table. Do for each grouping.

6. Add together the patients in "C" to obtain the projected shift census. Record in appropriate "Totals" box.

7. Add together the "Patient Care Hours" to obtain "Total Hours of Care" projected for the upcoming shift. Record in appropriate "Totals" box and "Total Patient Care Hours" box.

8. Divide by 8 to obtain the "Indicated Patient Care Givers" for that shift and record in appropriate box.

A new and closer working relationship among physicians, nurses, and administrators is essential.

ALTERNATIVE SYSTEMS

Alternative delivery systems are being created to afford entrepreneurial options for operational salvation and financial growth at traditional hospitals. Specialization is increasing among hospitals and particular services and diagnostic groups but basic reforms in the financing of hospital care may not. Prospective payment based on price and the reassignment of risk from payers to providers will continue, with modifications based on national data. Hospital decision making at the operational level is being altered to integrate clinical and administrative factors and to speed up the process with up-to-date information systems.

Long-range and strategic planning is receiving new emphasis with greater focus on program and service mixes. Organizational structures are being more product and management oriented. Mix strategy—vertical integration through diversification—and horizontal integration at least sufficient to allocate services is changing the management structure; both vertical and horizontal integrations require new corporate forms.

The American Organization of Nurse Executives 1985 guidelines on the role and functions of such individuals state that the "nurse executive participates in a systemwide assessment of management informational needs and the development of related policies and programs, including the establishment and maintenance of a suitable data base."[15] The challenge to develop and utilize information systems integrated in the clinical components of nursing care requires that nurse executives develop plans that are supported by appropriate resources for "an effective information system that facilitates and economizes clinical and management decision making, including the development of a nursing data base."

Nursing clinical and financial data are key in the entrepreneurial relationships. As noted in Chapter 6, the hospital research and educational trust used a grant funded by the W.K. Kellogg Foundation and the Duke Endowment to create a planning, budgeting, and clinical management system based on the integrated financial and clinical data streams of the hospital. It listed six data-related factors to be addressed:

1. quality of clinical data
2. quantity of data for operational analysis
3. methods for determining costs
4. integration of data streams
5. selection of appropriate definition of hospital product
6. comparability of information across hospitals.

APPLICABILITY TO NURSING

As financial pressures on hospitals increase, more data—both management and clinical—must be collected and analyzed. For example, answers are being sought for questions such as:

- How do the nurses' practice patterns relate to training, background, and specialty?
- Is there a difference between nurses with bachelor of science in nursing or master of science in nursing and nurses with other preparation?
- What is the health status of patients upon admission?
- What is the relative efficiency in a hospital's use of resources to produce a specific service?
- What are specific regional differences in case type?
- What are the differences in severity among patients with the same diagnosis?

Without detailed data, the clinician or manager is unable to assess the cause of a financial or quality variant, as stated in Chapter 1.

Marginal cost information is necessary when making financial decisions on adding or subtracting from the hospital's bottom line. Historically, the integration of clinical and financial data has been expensive and time consuming because of the large volumes of information involved. The surge in computer capacity has eliminated that factor as a problem. Large hospitals can afford computers with enough capacity to manage large data bases. The large data processing services can integrate data for hospitals that do not have their own computer capabilities. However, the software required for integrating clinical and financial data can be expensive to write.

Technical difficulties arise regarding unique patient identifiers for each data stream. These problems generally are solvable, particularly if the data are accurate. Existing systems may need to be refined for several reasons (see Chapter 1, pp. 8–9):

- Each was developed originally for a specific purpose.
- Each used a different patient population that might not totally reflect the client types found in a particular institution.
- Each was designed to explain other variables, such as length of stay or total charges, rather than a spectrum of resources allocated by hospital managers, nurses, and physicians.

Quality assurance data should focus on the validity of diagnostic and clinical information provided by the hospital. Factors involved include completeness, accuracy, quality of care, appropriateness of admissions and discharges, timeliness of discharge planning, and appropriateness of care for which additional payments are sought beyond the DRG rate. A clinical-financial information system can assist in this process by providing information on past utilization patterns for developing acceptable protocols and ranges of resource use. Identifying cases that fall outside the standard becomes both a nursing and a medical care mandate.

The medical record is insufficient as it exists. Nursing documentation is often inadequate in time and sequence of events. Nursing must develop information systems that integrate with it. Some of the factors limiting the record include (1) the quality of clinical data, so there will be no confidence in it; (2) the quantity of the clinical and financial data for defining clinical protocols and treatment. An integrated system must assist in the monitoring of quality care by the incorporation of existing clinical data streams such as nosocomial infection reports, pathology reports, incident reports, nursing risk management reports, current patient classification systems, and nursing quality assurance generic screens.

A key incentive for managers is to develop sound productivity measurements. They must pay greater attention to identifying and measuring the aggregation of hospital services and nursing required to produce the product. Productivity improvement is essential. Productivity comparisons in primary nursing indicate increased efficiency and reduction of costs while maintaining a level of quality commensurate with standards of practice.

Productivity measurements are illustrated in Figures 7–3 and 7–4. They demonstrate that primary nursing is more cost-efficient than nonprimary nursing. In a primary nursing environment, all nurses are providing direct care to each of their patients. Therefore, it is not necessary for them to spend time supervising or redoing the work of ancillary staff. Primary nursing is definitively more productive than nonprimary nursing. New measurement techniques and work methods must be combined with concern for two-way communication between nursing staff and management, staff motivation, and the work environment. An effective hospital productivity effort should involve all levels of nonmedical staff with management as well as with the medical staff.

Concerns of nursing staff for the quality of patient care must be addressed as crucial elements of any hospital productivity program. Quality assurance mechanisms need to be monitored and strengthened. Quality assurance computerized information systems for nursing are imperative. The role of physicians and nurses in hospital management decisions on productivity has not been too well defined in the past. Innovative models and methods for administration, medical staff, and nursing service collaboration and productivity issues need to be identified and evaluated.

Hospitals that cannot invest heavily in integrated data systems or shared systems will face serious problems. The new prospective payment system encourages the

Figure 7-3 Monthly Patient Day Trends

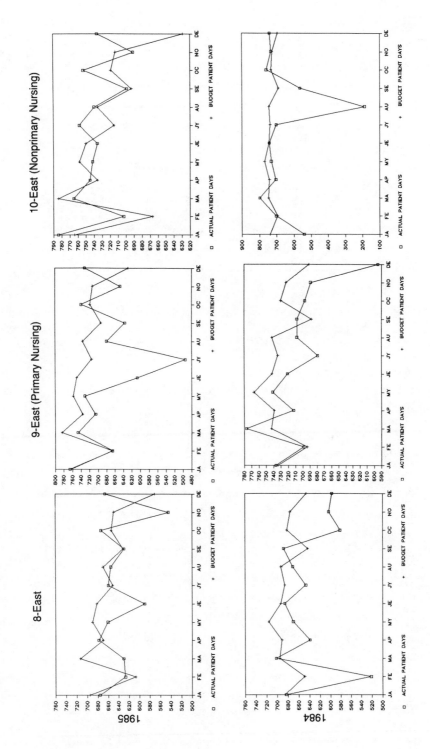

155

Figure 7–4 Monthly Productivity Trends

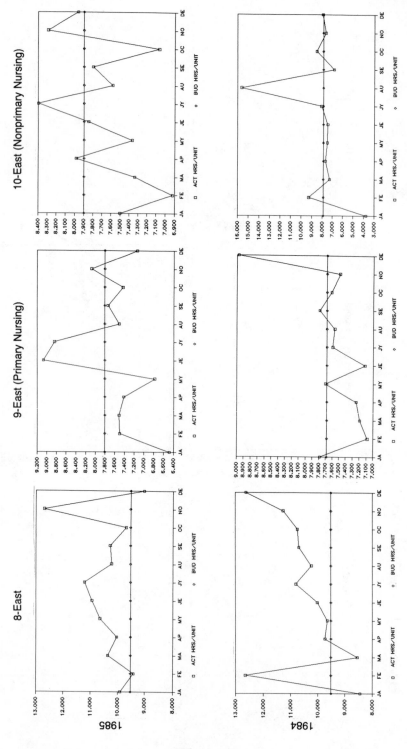

156

development of a three-tiered health care system based on ability to pay: One tier is self-insured plus ability to pay for all alternative treatment options; a second tier is HMO, PPO, and regular group insured; a third is Medicare/Medicaid and so-called "welfare." What forms this three-tier system might take and what effects it will have on the public as well as the nursing staff have yet to be determined.

The *Seattle Times* on April 22, 1985, carried an article "Health Care Becoming Stratified with the Poor at the Bottom." The article stressed new forces in health care financing as the beginning of limits on medical and hospital spending and how much government business and health insurers would pay doctors and hospitals. This trend is forcing almost all medical services to reassess how much care they will provide. This is affected by the explosion of new health care plans: HMOs, similar IPAs (doctors' independent practice associations), and the like. These take over all of their patients' medical and hospital care for a fixed monthly payment. A growing share of hospital medical care is being acquired by investor-owned profit-seeking businesses. The article points out that the striking fact about all three of these movements is that none has as its primary goal making patient care better.

In a *Medical Economics* article, Roger Russley, a Denver medical practice consultant, told doctors: "You will find the health care market breaking down into three classes, much as the airlines do: Class 1, for those who put the quality, comfort, and convenience of their health care above cost considerations. Class 2, for patients who consider cost first, so belong to an HMO or like plan where the choice of a physician will be somewhat limited. Class 3, for those covered by the government-subsidized plans like Medicare and Medicaid." More changes in health care are anticipated. Federal deficit levels and the fluctuating economy will force a regulatory framework that provides the right incentives for competition (e.g., free-standing "doc in the box" surgicenters as hospitals, etc.).

If DRGs are around by the early 1990s and other payers adopt the method, nursing systems need to be integrated strongly into it. If DRGs do not survive, another type of system (capitation) is likely to be the successor.

Financial managers of health care institutions will have to adopt new approaches. Nursing's ability to relate to integrated data systems that affect the management structures of health care settings must improve significantly if institutions are to prepare for these changes. It seems inevitable that hospitals will continue to remain financially vulnerable to decreased profit.

STRUCTURES UNDER THE NEW SYSTEM

New structures are being created to enable organizations to operate efficiently under the new payment system. The use of integrated data systems can change relationships among medical staff, boards of directors, and administration. Nursing must be part of those changes and assist with facilitating them through collaborative practice efforts. Barriers within organizations that block effective participation in clinical and financial data bases must be surmounted.

Whatever type and source of nursing information system is selected, it should permit nursing data to be linked to the existing data base. It is helpful to examine successful models in which integrated programs have been developed. Integrated data systems designed for prospective payments can affect the manner in which data such as the incidence of disease are recorded and could change the implications for epidemiological monitoring and research. The manner in which the data are recorded and collected will affect their accuracy, applicability, and compatibility from one nursing setting to another. Those committed to the application of information systems in nursing must develop a common data base that incorporates existing ones.

Most hospitals have quite complete management medical information systems, including comprehensive financial systems for patient accounting, general ledger, accounts payable, and payroll. Laboratories usually are equipped for data acquisition and comprehensive reporting of their results. Admitting data range from admissions, discharges, and transfers to patient registration, order communication, result reporting, appointments, and scheduling. Many hospital pharmacies have 24-hour service to supply information in an accumulative systems format. Medical records include abstracts, archival data, data analysis and reporting, interfacing with word processing systems between medical secretaries, surgical pathology, and administration. Nursing data needs include 24-hour staff scheduling, management information systems, patient classification systems, charting systems, patient discharge instructions, and general administrative capabilities such as nursing policies and procedures that allow flexibility and tailoring to meet specific needs.

The development and utilization of information systems integrated into clinical components of nursing care requires a comprehensive plan supported by appropriate resources for organizational effectiveness in an information system that facilitates clinical and managerial decision making.

NOTES

1. David B. Starkweather, "Organizational and Management Issues" (Paper delivered at the "Symposium on the Integration of Clinical and Financial Data Systems," Virginia Mason Foundation, Seattle, November 11–12, 1983).

2. President's Commission for the Study of Ethical Problems in Medicine and Biomedical and Behavioral Research, *Deciding to Forgo Life-Sustaining Treatment* (Washington, D.C.: U.S. Government Printing Office, March 1983).

3. Duane D. Walker, "Cost of Nursing Care in Hospitals," *Journal of Nursing Administration* (March 1983).

4. Ibid., 18.

5. Sovie, et al., "Amalgam of Nursing Acuity, DRG's and Costs," *Nursing Management* 16, no. 3 (March 1985).

6. Ibid., 41.

7. Ibid., 42.

8. Joint Commission on the Accreditation of Hospitals, *AMH/85* (Chicago: Author, 1984), 97.

9. Ibid., 98.

10. Calista Roy, *Introduction to Nursing: An Adaptation Model* (Englewood Cliffs, N.J.: Prentice-Hall, Inc., 1976), 20.

11. Nancy Higgerson and Ann Van Slyck, ''Variable Billing for Services: New Fiscal Direction for Nursing,'' *Journal of Nursing Administration* (June 1982).

12. Doris L. Carnevali, ''Nursing Perspectives in Health Care Technology,'' *Nursing Administration Quarterly* 9, no. 4 (Summer 1985), 10–18.

13. _____, *Nursing Care Planning: Diagnosis and Management,* 3rd edition (Philadelphia: J.B. Lippincott Co., 1983).

14. Harriet Werley, ''Proceedings of the Postconference Task Force Meeting on the Nursing Minimum Data Set (NMDS)'' (Paper delivered at the Nursing Minimum Data Sets Conference, University of Wisconsin-Milwaukee, September 1985).

15. ''Role and Functions of the Hospital Nurse Executive,'' *American Hospital Association Guidelines,* No. 054700, 12M/5-85-1071 (Chicago: AHA, 1985).

Appendix 7–A

Additional Patient Classification Systems

ICU PATIENT CLASSIFICATION SYSTEM

M ICU PATIENT CLASSIFICATION FORM
VIRGINIA MASON HOSPITAL

DATE _____
REPORT PREPARED BY _____
SHIFT   Day for Evening ( ), Evening for Night ( ), Night for Day ( )

1-11 ICU-NO _____
12-23 ICU-SO _____

CENSUS _____
PEND. ADMIT. Heart _____ Other _____
PEND. DISCH. _____

	PATIENT CARE NEEDS	
PHYSIOLOGICAL MONITORING	Vital Signs (T.P.R.BP)	A
	Neuro Checks	B
	Arterial Reading	C
	Swan Ganz Reading	D
	CVP Reading	E
	Cardiac Output/SVR	F
	ICP Reading	G
	API Reading	H
	Postural BP & P	I
	Intake and Output	J
	Pedal Pulses	K
	Abdominal Girth	L
	Chest Tube Stripping and Reading	M
RESPIRATORY MONITORING	ET/NT Suction	N
	CDB/Respirex	O
	Bennett/Nebulized Meds	P
	Turn with Nurse Assist	Q
MENTAL STATUS	Alert/Coorperative	A
	Obtunded/Lethargic	B
	Confused/Restrained	C
ISOLATION	HW/Resp/Bl/St/Ur	D
	Protective/Standard	E
	Dressing Isolation	F
CARDIO-VASCULAR MANAGEMENT	Cardiac Monitoring	G
	Pacemaker on/Freq. Arrhy	H
	Swan Ganz	I
	Arterial Line	J
	TEDS/Ace Wraps	K
	Actively Bleeding	L
	IABP	M
SOCIOCULTURAL	Sp. Communication Needs of Pt/Family	N
	Discharge/Transfer	O

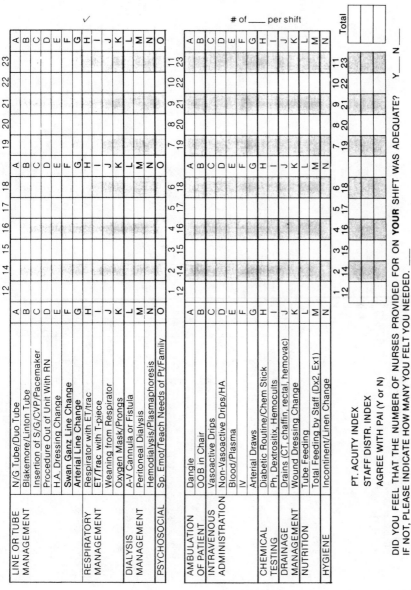

		12 14	14 15	15 16	16 17	17 18	18	19	20	21	22 23		
LINE OR TUBE MANAGEMENT	N/G Tube/Duo Tube	A										A	
	Blakemore/Linton Tube	B										B	
	Insertion of S/G/CVP/Pacemaker	C										C	
	Procedure Out of Unit With RN	D										D	
	H.A. Dressing Change	E										E	
	Swan Ganz Line Change	F										F	
	Arterial Line Change	G										G	
RESPIRATORY MANAGEMENT	Respirator with ET/trac	H										H	
	ET/Trac with T-piece	I										I	
	Weaning from Respirator	J										J	
	Oxygen Mask/Prongs	K										K	
DIALYSIS MANAGEMENT	A-V Cannula or Fistula	L										L	
	Peritoneal Dialysis	M										M	
	Hemodialysis/Plasmaphoresis	N										N	
PSYCHOSOCIAL	Sp. Emot/Teach Needs of Pt/Family	O										O	

# of ____ per shift

		1 12	2 14	3 15	4 16	5 17	6 18	7 19	8 20	9 21	10 22	11 23		
AMBULATION OF PATIENT	Dangle	A											A	
	OOB in Chair	B											B	
INTRAVENOUS ADMINISTRATION	Vasoactive Drips	C											C	
	Non-Vasoactive Drips/HA	D											D	
	Blood/Plasma	E											E	
	IV	F											F	
	Arterial Draws	G											G	
CHEMICAL TESTING	Diabetic Routine/Chem Stick	H											H	
	Ph. Dextrositix, Hemocults	I											I	
DRAINAGE MANAGEMENT	Drains (CT, chaffin, rectal, hemovac)	J											J	
	Wound Dressing Change	K											K	
NUTRITION	Tube Feeding	L											L	
	Total Feeding by Staff (Dx2, Ex1)	M											M	
HYGIENE	Incontinent/Linen Change	N											N	

Total

PT. ACUITY INDEX

STAFF DISTR. INDEX

AGREE WITH PAI (Y or N)

DID YOU FEEL THAT THE **NUMBER OF NURSES** PROVIDED FOR ON **YOUR** SHIFT WAS ADEQUATE?   Y___ N___

IF NOT, PLEASE INDICATE HOW MANY YOU FELT YOU NEEDED. ___

CCU PATIENT CLASSIFICATION SYSTEM

Date _____
Report prepared by _____
Shift - Day for Evening ( ), Evening for Night ( ), Night for Day ( )

**M CCU PATIENT CLASSIFICATION FORM
VIRGINIA MASON HOSPITAL**

PATIENT CARE NEEDS		WEIGHT	1	2	3	4	5	6	7	8
NURSING ASSESSMENT	1 V/S (T,P,BP)	1 x 1								
	2 EKG taken by RN	2								
CARDIAC PAIN	3 Unstable Type A	9								
	4 Unstable Type B	6								
	5 Stable	3								
NON CARDIAC PAIN	6 Uncontrolled	2								
	6 Controlled	1								
MEDICATION ADMINISTRATION	8 IV Infusion/Bolus - Type A	1 x 7								
	9 IV Infusion/Bolus - Type B	1 x 5								
	10 IV/PO Medication	1 x 2								
	11 Routine/IV/prn/PO Medication	1 x 1								
	12 IV Monitoring	1 x 1								
INVASIVE TECHNIQUES/ HEMODYNAMIC MONITORING	SET-UP, INSERTION AND CLEAN-UP									
	13 Swan-Ganz	7								
	14 Swan-Ganz C-arm	9								
	15 Temporary Pacemaker	8								
	16 Arterial Line	4								
	REPOSITIONING									
	17 Swan-Ganz	3								
	18 Swan-Ganz with C-arm	5								
	19 Temporary Pacemaker	5								
	READING, CALIBRATING, STIMULATION THRESHOLD:									
	20 Swan-Ganz	1 + 3								
	21 Temporary Pacer	1								
	22 Arterial Line	1 + 3								
	23 Cardiac Output	1 x 2								
	TUBING & DRESSING CHANGE									
	24 Swan-Ganz	3								
	25 Temporary Pacemaker	1								
	26 Arterial Line	3								
	27 Arterial Line Blood Draw	1 x 1								

Calculation Area

Σ PCH ÷ 8 = _____ Patient Care Providers

_____ Ward Secretary

_____ Required Staff

SCHEDULED STAFF

	Days		Evenings		Nights	
NCC	RN		RN		RN	
	Plus	-W.S.	Plus	-W.S.	Plus	-W.S.

	ACUITY CLASS			TOTAL NUMBER OF PATIENTS
	1:3	1:2	1:1	
NUMBER OF PATIENTS				

Did you feel that the number of nurses provided on **your shift** was adequate? Y ___ N ___

If not, how many? _____ please explain why.

Comment:

Do you feel that the predicted staffing for the **oncoming**

Shift is adequate? Y ___ N ___

If not, how many? _____ please explain why.

Comment:

RESPIRATORY	28	ET Tube and Ventilation	3									
	29	ET Tube and T-Piece	2									
	30	Nasal Prongs/Mask	1									
	31	Suctioning	1 x 1									
	32	Cough & DB/Respirex	1 x 1									
PHYSICAL CARE	33	Complete Bed Bath	4									
	34	Partial Bed Bath	3									
	35	Nurse Assisted Turning & Repositioning	1 x 1									
	36	Cath Care	1									
	37	Enemas	2									
	38	DR & Chem Strips	1 x 1									
	39	N/G Maintenance	2									
	40	Nausea and Vomiting	2									
	41	Foley	1 x 1									
PATIENT TEACHING/PSYCH		PSYCH SUPPORT/TEACHING										
	42	Days	3									
	43	Evenings	4									
	44	Nights	3									
	45	Pre-op Teaching	2									
	46	Post Heart Cath Teaching	3									
	47	Special Emotional Needs	*									
TRANSFERS	48	X-Ray	4									
	49	Echo	5									
	50	Heart Cath Lab	4									
	51	Surgery	3									
	52	PVP	6									
	53	Lung Scan	8									
	54	MUGA	-									
	55	Discharge/Transfer										
	56	Other										
SOCIO CULTURAL	57	Communication Bar										
	58	Special Dietary Nee										
SPIRITUAL	59	Spiritual Comfort for										
MENTAL STATUS	60	Confused										
	61	Restraints & Obser										
	62	Continual Observati										
CODE	63	Code 4 Alert										
	64	24 Hour Post Code										
UNIT CONSTANT												
SHIFT CO-EFFICIENT D												
E												
N												
ACUITY SCORE												
PATIENT CARE HOURS												
Agree with Acuity Class? (Y or N)												

CONVERSION TABLE

Acuity Class	1:3	1:2	1:1
Acuity Score	<30	>30-70	>70
Patient Care Hours	2.5	4	8.0

FM379 3/82

REHABILITATION PATIENT CLASSIFICATION SYSTEM

M REHABILITATION PATIENT CLASSIFICATION FORM
VIRGINIA MASON HOSPITAL

Date _____
Report prepared by _____
Staffing prediction for DAYS( ) EVENINGS( ) NIGHTS( )

Calculation Area

PATIENT CARE NEEDS		Wts	1	2	3	4	5	6	7	8	9	10	11	12
FEEDING	1. Minimal Assist (D × 2, E × 1)	1.f												
	2. Moderate Assist (D × 2, E × 1)	3.f												
	3. Maximum Assist (D × 2, E × 1)	5.f												
	4. Structured Fluid Intake Regime	3												
GROOMING (Face, Hair, Teeth, Shaving)	5. Minimal Assist	1												
	6. Moderate Assist	3												
	7. Maximum Assist	5												
BATHING (Bed, Shower, Tub)	8. Minimal Assist	2												
	9. Moderate Assist	4												
	10. Maximum Assist	5												
DRESSING/UNDRESSING (Upper Extremity-Includes clothing and sling)	11. Minimal Assist	2												
	12. Moderate Assist	2												
	13. Maximum Assist	3												
DRESSING/UNDRESSING (Lower Extremity-Includes clothing, shoes, socks, braces)	14. Minimal Assist	1												
	15. Moderate Assist	2												
	16. Maximum Assist	3												
BOWEL MANAGEMENT	17. Minimal Assist	3.f												
	18. Moderate Assist	4.f												
	19. Maximum Assist	5.f												
BLADDER MANAGEMENT	20. Minimal Assist	1.f												
	21. Moderate Assist	3.f												
	22. Maximum Assist	4.f												
MOBILITY (Bed)	23. Minimal Assist	1.f												
	24. Moderate Assist	2.f												
	25. Maximum Assist	3.f												
	26. Range of Motion	2												

Σ PCH ÷ 8 = _____ Patient Care Providers

SCHEDULED STAFF

	Days			Evening			Nights	
	NCC	RN	LPN	NCC	RN	LPN	RN	LPN

Plus ___ W.S. Plus ___ W.S. Plus
___ N.A. ___ N.A.

	ACUITY CLASS			TOTAL NUMBER OF PATIENTS
	.5	I	II	III
NUMBER OF PATIENTS				

Did you feel that the number of nurses provided on **your** shift was adequate? Y ___ N ___

If not, how many needed ? ___ please explain why.

Comment: _____

Do you feel that the predicted staffing for the
oncoming shift is adequate? Y ____ N ____
If not, how many needed? ____ please explain why.
Comment:

CONVERSION TABLE

Acuity Class	.5	I	II	III
Acuity Score	≤10	11-20	21-50	≥51
Patient Care Hours	.5	1	2	3

Category	Item	Value
TRANSFERS	27. Minimal Assist	1.f
	28. Moderate Assist	2.f
	29. Maximum Assist	3.f
	30. Ambulation	2.f
INTEGUMENT	31. Pressure Management	3
	32. Skin Care	2.f
	33. Wound Care	2.f
SAFETY	34. Minimal Supervision	4
	35. Moderate Supervision	5
	36. Maximum Supervision	6
ALTERNATE COMMUNICATION SYSTEM - 37.		5
ASSESSMENT PARAMETERS	38. Vital Signs (BP, P, T)	1.f
	39. Postural BPs	1.f
	40. Intake and Output	1.f
	41. Weights	1
	42. Chemstrips	1.f
	43. Specimens - Collection and Testing	1.f
IV AND MED ADMINISTRATION	44. Difficult PO/Insulin	1.f
	45. IV/Partial Fill	2.f
	46. SAM (Self-Administration of Medication)	1.f
PAIN MANAGEMENT/BEHAVIOR MODIFICATION PROGRAM	47. Baseline	6
	48. Treatment	5
PATIENT/FAMILY COUNSELING - 49.		4.f
SPECIAL ACTIVITIES - 50.		5.f
SPIRITUAL	51. Spiritual Comfort for Pt./Family	2
SOCIO-CULTURAL	52. Adjustment to Cultural Variations	3
DISCHARGE PLANNING	53. Intake Evaluation	6
	54. Patient/Family Conferences	5
	55. Home Care Arrangements	3
	56. Referrals	5
	57. Discharge	5
	58. Unit Constant	3
ACUITY SCORE		
PATIENT CARE HOURS		
AGREE WITH ACUITY CLASS? (Y or N)		

FM 395-484

Chapter 8

Information Systems for Decision Support: Hospital Census Management

Vandan Trivedi

The onset of the 1980s saw the health care industry enter an era of marketplace competition. The inception of prospective reimbursement based on diagnosis related groups (DRGs) for Medicare patients in October 1983 introduced yet another major change in the dynamics of the industry. Hospital occupancies and patient lengths of stay promptly began to decline. On the other hand, ambulatory surgeries and ambulatory visits are on the rise. To maintain their share of the eroding inpatient base, hospitals now are openly competing against each other.

This is a major turning point in the health care industry. Hospitals are beginning to operate like any other business entity, with careful consideration of reducing costs, increasing efficiency and productivity, and maintaining a quality level of their product—patient care. DRG-based prospective reimbursement has significant ramifications in that hospitals are becoming more selective in the kinds of patients they will admit; admissions of cases in DRGs that lose money are discouraged.

Under the twin forces of competition and regulation, the task of management in the health care industry is becoming even more challenging. Conventional tools and techniques of business management—marketing, strategic planning, financial modeling, decision support systems—heretofore uncommon in this industry are becoming commonplace. As these major changes are occurring, information and computer technology in the industry also are undergoing a major revolution, with enormous impact. This results from the fact that there are few industries that are so information-dependent and in which such large groups of diverse professionals work together.

During the 1960s and 1970s, a majority of hospitals installed conventional hospital information systems that included patient billing and accounts receivable, admitting, registration, discharges and transfers, laboratory, pharmacy, and materials management. These systems, in most instances, are housed in time-shared mainframe computers with terminals spread around various hospital departments.

The systems typically are maintained and serviced by hospital data processing departments.

THE THRUST FOR INTEGRATION

However, the 1980s have seen a change in this modus operandi. The regulations have made it necessary to integrate clinical and financial information systems. There are new demands on those systems for target marketing of hospital services, for developing competitive pricing structures, for better patient care, and for improved resource allocation. Advances in medical technology such as computerized axial tomography (CT) scanners, magnetic resonance (MR) imaging, and critical care patient monitoring also have put unique demands on hospital information systems, requiring digital imaging networks (DINs) and sophisticated computerized telecommunications.

The role of conventional data processing departments in hospitals also is changing drastically. The so-called ''data processing function'' increasingly is distributed throughout the hospital. Clinicians, managers, and technicians are designing their own systems and user interfaces rather than relying exclusively on data processing departments. The advent of user-friendly fourth-generation languages is making it possible for noncomputer experts to communicate with computers in plain English-like languages to design and customize their individual requirements. The role of a conventional data processing department is becoming more defused throughout the hospital and is evolving into the new role of an information center. The primary responsibility of an information center is to assume leadership in assisting and training users throughout the hospital and leading them in the right direction vis-a-vis their information needs.

During the 1960s and 1970s, computers were applied almost entirely to clerical tasks and repetitive transaction processing. However, in the 1980s, this area has focused on decision support systems to help managers in their decision-making activities such as analysis, planning, resource allocation, forecasting, and reporting. These represent tasks in which human judgment joined with automation can be more effective than either by itself. Decision support systems have become, in a short time, an established part of an organization's computing resources.

This chapter analyzes the impact of advances in information systems on management decision support systems in hospitals. A decision support system designed for managing hospital census variations is used to illustrate this impact. This system has been implemented in several hospitals.

CENSUS MANAGEMENT SYSTEM (CMS)

The census management system (CMS) is a decision support method that melds human judgment with a computerized information system. Typical decision questions that need to be addressed are: how many patients to schedule, how many beds to have available for emergencies, whether to transfer a patient to another unit, and if the census is low, whether to close a unit. Instead of describing the technical aspects of the system, this chapter looks at the general concepts underlying the system and its implications for hospitals operating in different environments.

Faced with lower occupancies and higher operating costs, some hospitals are considering unit closures. They are thinking creatively about meeting the needs and preferences of their patient and physician populations. To strike a balance between the ever-increasing cost of nurse staffing, on the one hand, and maintaining an acceptable level of care, on the other, appropriate placement of patients on nursing units has become very important. Even the Joint Commission on the Accreditation of Hospitals has stated clearly in its 1985 manual that "the hospital admissions system should allow for input from the nursing department/service in coordinating patient requirements for nursing care with available nursing resources."[1]

In essence, the census management system consists of developing various benchmarks and guidelines on a computer-based simulation model.[2,3] These are designed for daily use by the admitting officer, patient placement nurse, or surgery scheduler. The guidelines address such issues as the number of surgical and medical patients to schedule on various days, the number of beds to keep open for emergency admissions on each unit, the optimum census level for each unit, etc. The computer model develops these guidelines by incorporating historical data on lengths of stay, admissions, discharges, transfers, surgery schedules, and other factors. The person in charge of census management (usually a patient placement nurse) integrates the guidelines for making admission, transfer, and patient placement decisions.

Although the system is relatively straightforward, for successful operation it needs cooperation from admitting physicians; therefore, from the very beginning, their active participation is sought. They are educated in the concepts underlying the system, and the fact that their admission practices have tremendous impact on the hospital census is impressed on them. They also are made aware of the fact that in order to (1) be able to place their patients on the most appropriate nursing units, (2) always have an adequate number of beds available for emergency admissions, (3) stabilize the hospital census (and hence the workload) and (4) not cause inconvenience or delay to them and their patients, it is necessary that they understand the system and honor the guidelines. The system has benefits for physicians as well as for their patients.

The overall system consists of several components, all of which must be implemented for a successful operation: a system of classifying emergency, urgent, and elective patients; a system of scheduling medical and surgical patients; and the establishment of a physician committee to monitor the operation. Once all the components are in place, the system controls daily admissions of elective and urgent patients while allowing immediate admission of emergencies.

SYSTEM BENEFITS

It takes six to nine months to collect all the information, analyze the data, run the computer model, train the hospital personnel, and finally implement the system. Once it is in place, several concrete benefits become obvious. The most important is stable occupancy and better utilization of hospital beds. Since hospitals have an extremely large fixed cost of operation per bed, it is crucial to distribute those fixed costs efficiently over a large proportion of patients by improving bed utilization. Stable occupancy means a predictable workload not only for nursing service but also for other ancillary departments such as admitting, laboratory, radiology, dietary, and pharmacy. This also eliminates the need for adding beds during peak census.

The system provides the admitting department with objectivity in planning admissions and transfers and in predicting future census. It also facilitates patient placement on the most appropriate units. Operating room utilization is improved, and communication among physicians, patient placement, admitting, and surgery is enhanced. The system acts as a catalyst for reducing work-related stress and elevating morale in admitting, surgery, and nursing units.

With better bed utilization, hospitals can reduce or postpone expansion needs, which has the potential for large savings in operating and capital costs. Because of lower variation in census, hospital staffing costs are reduced, since the standby staffing and overtime required to meet peak loads in every department are significantly less. Fewer transfers also imply savings in housekeeping and nursing.

COMPETITION AMONG HOSPITALS

As noted, every hospital faces some level of competition for patients. However, the degree of competition varies according to the services the hospital offers, its location, the type of medical staff, and other factors. At one extreme, a hospital could face minimum competition and run at quite high occupancies, while at the other extreme it could face fierce competition and have low occupancies. Of course, there are numerous hospitals that operate anywhere between those two extremes. The CMS is applicable in each environment, but there are significant differences in the strategy of implementation of the system, as discussed next.

High Occupancy and Low Competition

A hospital with high occupancy (say, medical/surgical occupancy of 85 percent and above) experiences a severe bed crunch from time to time. Usually the waiting period for elective surgery in such a hospital is quite long (six to eight weeks); at times no beds will be available for emergency admissions and the hospital may have to create extra beds or even divert patients to a nearby hospital.

Because of the extremely high demand for beds, it may not be possible to place all patients on the most appropriate nursing units and this could lead to an increase in the number of transfers. This produces more tension and dissatisfaction among employees, especially in admitting, nursing, and surgery; there usually is an increase in patient, physician, and employee complaints as well.

The census management system is extremely effective under these circumstances in alleviating the hospital's bed-related problems and in relieving employee tension. By stabilizing variations and increasing the mean occupancy, the system in effect "creates" additional beds instantaneously. Since in this situation the physicians normally do not object to putting their patients on a wait list, provided it will guarantee an earlier admission, the hospital can use that list to its advantage in reducing the valleys in census.

A hospital experiencing high demand wants to fill every available bed as soon as possible. This happens to be consistent with physicians' objectives of expeditiously acquiring beds for their patients. Therefore, physicians do not mind if occasionally their patients are not placed on the most appropriate nursing units. For example, an orthopedic patient may be placed on a general medical/surgical unit, provided the case is an urgent one and no orthopedic beds are open. With its need to maintain high occupancy, the hospital certainly takes a higher risk of turning away emergency patients or rescheduling elective surgeries. However, after carefully weighing all the alternatives, it can decide at what level of risk it can afford to operate.

Because of the low competition environment, the hospital has greater latitude in achieving its objectives and in working with physicians. Nevertheless, the hospital must have a great deal of cooperation from physicians if it is to implement CMS successfully. Their cooperation is needed to ensure that they do not abuse the system and also to mediate with peers in conflict situations.

Low Occupancy and High Competition

For a hospital experiencing low occupancy in a highly competitive market, the CMS can be an effective tool for making sure that the facility does not lose patients to other institutions and that patients always are placed on the most appropriate nursing unit, where they can receive optimum care of consistently high quality. The CMS guidelines can be so designed that individual preferences of physicians can be fulfilled. By reducing census variations, the system not only enables a hospital to reduce staffing costs but also provides the stable staffing necessary for high quality care.

In implementing the system, cooperation from physicians is sought to determine when they make rounds, when they prefer to do surgery, what their days off are, what their admitting habits are, etc. This information can be obtained through a questionnaire survey, with the results incorporated into the system.

Before implementing the system, the census variation in low-occupancy hospitals is even greater than in high-occupancy hospitals. This is because the natural limit of bed capacity prevents a high-occupancy hospital census from taking large swings. In a low-occupancy hospital, the bed capacity ceiling is much higher, so the census shows larger variations. An important role of CMS in such hospitals is maintaining the census of each unit within an occupancy frame consistent with the unit's nurse staffing.

In this situation, because of the possibility that wait-listed patients could be diverted to other hospitals, there is less emphasis on putting them on such a list. Similarly, the system is designed to eliminate chances of elective surgery cancellation and emergency turnaways, thus guaranteeing timely admission to all patients. The scheduling guidelines in such a hospital are not used for denying admissions but merely for a benchmark against which actual patient demand can be monitored.

To reduce costs, a hospital may even consider closing some beds. But, unless objective criteria are available, it is difficult to make this decision. The system can be of great assistance in determining precisely how many beds to close and when to do so. It provides specific census levels and admission/discharge forecasts as objective criteria for each unit. When the census of a unit falls below a predetermined level and the admission/discharge forecast does not meet the criteria, the hospital should close that unit. The system thus plays a significant role in providing optimum care, in reducing costs, in satisfying physician preferences, and most importantly in ascertaining that the hospital does not lose patients to other facilities.

DIFFERENCES AMONG HOSPITALS

Just as the environment of a hospital needs special consideration, so does the type of hospital. Since 1980, the author has implemented the system in a variety of hospitals, including a university-based teaching hospital, a pediatric hospital, a health maintenance organization (HMO) hospital, and a community general hospital. As discussed next, each type of hospital has unique requirements that must be incorporated into its census management system for successful implementation.

A university-based hospital must meet the special teaching needs of its faculty, medical students, and residents. This normally implies that a specific number of beds on each nursing unit are allocated to each specialty and subspecialty.

However, adhering to a fixed bed quota within each unit is counterproductive as far as overall bed utilization is concerned. Because of the random nature of patient demand, it is virtually impossible to control census within the strict boundaries specified by such quotas. The CMS is useful in improving bed utilization within the constraints of hospitals' teaching needs. Moreover, teaching hospitals experience a large number of patient transfers because of their numerous specialty units. The system also is instrumental in reducing the number of transfers, because specific guidelines are provided for scheduling and placement of patients, based on historical demand. These guidelines are developed to minimize the number of transfers.

Pediatric hospitals have a special requirement in that patients must be placed according to specific age groups. Normally infants, toddlers, and teenagers are segregated in different units. The separation is necessary not only for the patients' welfare but also because of the specialized nature of the nursing care. Another important consideration is the need for a large proportion of isolation beds. It is not uncommon for a pediatric hospital to have 20 to 30 percent of its patients in isolation beds on any given day. Patient placement policies are developed in CMS using historical age distributions of patients and their isolation requirements. These policies, when used in practice, facilitate meeting the age group and isolation bed demand. It is crucial, however, to analyze carefully the patient demand by age group and by isolation requirements, and to integrate this information into the system.

Hospitals owned by HMOs also have unique census management requirements. These facilities do not have any incentives to increase hospitalization among their enrollee populations since it is relatively more expensive to treat a patient in a hospital. Nevertheless, the HMO hospitals must avoid long backlogs of elective surgeries as well as excessive delays in admissions for fear of bad publicity. Further, these hospitals must reduce costs by improving utilization and controlling staffing. They must avoid having their patients diverted to non-HMO hospitals because they lack beds, since it is more expensive to purchase hospital services from outside. With carefully customizing the system to the hospital utilization characteristics of an HMO's subscribers, it can be instrumental in achieving an HMO's objectives.

The CMS also plays a significant role in a fee-for-service community general hospital. This type of hospital has to meet the needs of its patient population and attending physicians. Reducing daily variation in census enables such a hospital to provide consistent nurse staffing and to place patients on the most appropriate units. An important effect of reducing census fluctuations is felt in the operating rooms, in that their workload is stabilized. This is desired not only by the operating room nursing staff but also by anesthesiologists.

In summary, a census management system is an effective tool for optimum utilization of hospital resources, including beds, nursing staff, operating rooms, and ancillary services. The system facilitates providing more timely and improved services to patients and physicians. It significantly contributes to a hospital's efforts in cost reduction and improving quality of care. However, the system must be tailored to the specific requirements of each institution and, more importantly, the strategy of implementing the system must be uniquely designed for each hospital by incorporating patient, physician, and nursing staff preferences and the hospital's admitting and scheduling policies.

DECISION SUPPORT SYSTEMS

Several generalizations may be drawn from this paradigm in applying it to the development and implementation of decision support systems in a health care environment:

- Decision support is the specific application of available and appropriate technology to managerial tasks. In this chapter, the system addresses as an example the managerial tasks of reducing daily census variations, providing consistent quality and quantity of nursing resources, and improving utilization of hospital resources.
- The aim of a decision support system is to support, not to automate, decision making. The decisions as to whether to admit, when to admit, or onto which unit to admit constitute an extremely complex activity and require the joint assessment of several professionals. What the CMS has accomplished is to provide appropriate and timely information to a manager based on historical data to assist in decision making.
- Decision support systems must be easy to learn and use, responsive and flexible. This requires an adaptive design process by which complex systems are evolved out of simple components. It is important that the system adapt to the user, not vice versa. In the CMS example, physicians, nurses, and managers find it very easy to understand the basic premise of the system.
- A decision support system can represent major organizational and cultural change, and its implementation has to go well beyond installing a technical solution. In the CMS implementation, it is necessary to make allowances for behavioral changes of physicians, nurses, and managers. If the implementation process does not include appropriate training of these key players, the system could be perceived as a threat and they will refuse to use it. However, if the system implementer carefully trains and orients key players, they will be ardent supporters. The implementer needs to be a hybrid—fluent about the application and literate about the technical tools.

In conclusion, hospitals offer a rich environment for development and implementation of various decision support systems in several key management functions. These include finance, strategic planning, marketing, staff scheduling, patient scheduling, and operating room scheduling. Hospitals definitely feel there is a need for support on such decisions. An increasing number of decision support systems are being made available to hospitals, but their success will depend on how well their designers and implementers adapt to the unique environment of health care facilities.

NOTES

1. *Accreditation Manual for Hospitals* (Chicago: Joint Commission on the Accreditation of Hospitals, 1985), p. 98.
2. V.M. Trivedi and W.M. Hancock, "Tripartite Approach to Hospital Census Management," *Hospital and Health Services Administration* 26, special issue I (November 1981): 8–25.
3. V.M. Trivedi, M.J. Lee, and J. Hess, "Managing Hospital Census with Physician and Administration Teamwork," *Hospital and Health Services Administration* 30, no. 3 (May/June 1985): 58–71.

Chapter 9

Integrated Data Systems: The Research and the Future Agenda

Douglas A. Conrad

This chapter, a discussion and synthesis of research on integrated data systems, more fundamentally addresses a new technology in the health services industry. That is, data systems and management information systems that integrate clinical and financial information actually constitute a technological innovation. The innovation in this case is the combination of a managerially relevant and clinically coherent patient-mix classification scheme with financial information historically of primary interest to the management side of the health care enterprise.

As in any technological innovation, research in this area must address both its adoption and its utilization. Thus, the discussion of research on integrated data systems focuses here on those that have been adopted by health care organizations and how they have been used.

The research on integrated data systems has not used this taxonomy—either the distinction between managerial relevance and clinical coherence of the data system and underlying patient mix classification, or the notion of examining and evaluating which factors contribute specifically to its adoption and use as a new technology. Nonetheless, these distinctions are useful and serve to focus on a research agenda that is of immediate interest to administrators, physicians, information systems specialists and analysts, third party payers, and the research community itself.

OVERVIEW OF THE RESEARCH

In surveying the research on integrated clinical and financial data systems, the author has perceived two broad kinds of work:

1. descriptions of systems in use, with a heavy focus on case-based cost accounting

179

2. conceptual discussions and empirical comparisons of different integrated data systems (often concentrating on the underlying case-mix classification mechanism), including analyses of the utilization of integrated data for reporting, planning, budgeting, and controlling; the design of alternative case-mix classification schemas; and analyses of case-specific cost-accounting methodologies.

The descriptive work on systems in use is well represented by the writings of Burik and Duvall,[1] Bisbee and McCarthy,[2] and Corn.[3] The Burik and Duvall article describes hospital costing software and discusses the process of developing standard costs, not only for broad case-mix classifications such as diagnosis related groups (DRGs) but also for specific service items within a given cost center. The focus of that research is on a descriptive presentation of alternative methods of standard costing. In a separate work,[4] Burik and Duvall go on to discuss a range of approaches to standard costing, ranging from the use of simple ratios of cost to charge (RCC) to the standard bill of services.

Much of the case-based cost-accounting literature concentrates on the development of three kinds of systems:

1. stand-alone case-mix software, which typically allows management to provide cost-to-charge ratios at the department or cost center level, then uses these RCCs to produce cost estimates
2. patient costing systems that permit standard cost estimates to be derived at the level of the specific service item, which then can be reaggregated into standard costs per DRG or per other case type classification desired by the user
3. standard bill of service systems that develop detailed costs for materials, labor, and overhead for a single unit of a single service.

An important focus of the literature represented by Burik and Duvall is the discussion of how such case-specific costing systems might be used in reporting and in controlling behavior.[5] For example, this looks at the identification of different types of variances between actual and budgeted (predicted) costs as a result of price and activity factors believed to be at least partly within the control of the administrator and/or clinician.

Another element on systems in use is described by Bisbee and McCarthy,[6] who present a system for planning, budgeting, and controlling within the context of a health maintenance organization (HMO). They analyze the types of reports that an integrated data system might produce for a population-based health delivery system. Rounding out the descriptive work is a strand of research represented by Corn[7] that summarizes the impact of data errors on reimbursement for hospital services. This line of inquiry stresses the effect of errors in diagnostic coding, surgical procedure coding, and other issues related to the quality of data abstracted from the medical record on the average level of payment for services per hospital episode.

Generally, this research is concentrated on whether or not such errors lead to biases—either upward or downward—on the level of payment received in relation to the actual underlying cost of a hospital episode. A separate question generally not addressed involves the implications of such data errors for accurate reporting by specific diagnoses. The research has tended to select one or two sample diagnoses, not chosen for their representativeness, as illustrations of the impact such data errors might have on reimbursement. The same literature is oriented toward the inpatient hospital setting: to the extent ambulatory care case-based integrated data systems are considered, the impact of data errors in coding a given patient or episode on payment or other management or clinical outcomes has not been included in the analysis.[8,9]

The conceptual and empirical (as compared with descriptive) research on integrated data systems, represented by the work of Young and Saltman,[10] Griffith,[11] and Steinwachs,[12] has highlighted the importance of integrated data systems for four administrative purposes: reporting, planning, budgeting, and controlling.

Young and Saltman emphasize the need for a wholly different outlook on managerial control in the context of case-based prospective reimbursement for hospital care. Their thesis essentially is that data for managerial control need to be matched to the variables that an individual decision maker can control. Thus, in the context of the case-based data system, they stress the importance of designing a continuing reporting and controlling mechanism that provides special information to physicians, midlevel managers, and top management, respectively.

Griffith's early work (1976) addressed the criteria and procedures for setting up accounting control systems. While not focusing on integrated data systems per se, in the sense of case-mix classification linked to financial data, he does summarize an important set of considerations for designing an integrated data system:

- controlling costs
- strengthening the existing management structure
- emphasizing major cost components for management and clinical performance
- encouraging supervisory participation
- simplifying calculations and improving responsibility center management understanding
- dealing with variability in hospital activity
- stimulating continued improvement.

Griffith also describes a process of developing a budgeting and control system that dovetails nicely with the later work of Burik and Duvall (1985) that relates more explicitly to case-based, integrated data systems.

In an important 1985 contribution, Steinwachs describes an integrated ambulatory care management information system that links patient registration information with provider identification and a record unique to each visit (encounter). That kind of conceptualization is important in generalizing what has been primarily hospital-oriented information systems development to the ambulatory care and population-based systems.

An important series of articles addresses the design of case-mix classification systems.[13,14] This research on alternative patient classification methodologies does not connect patient clinical and financial information directly with data systems, but it cannot be separated from the design of integrated data systems. Horn and Schumacher[13] compare three schema for patient-mix classification and analyze the power of each of those systems in explaining variations in charges and length of stay at the level of the individual hospital episode. They find that a severity of illness index enhances the usefulness of the case-mix information present in the DRG and Patient Management category measures of case mix. Gonnella[14] extends the analysis by targeting the significance of constructing case-mix categories that are clinically meaningful, arguing both theoretically and empirically that such clinical coherence is helpful in data systems that attempt to explain behavior (cost, charges, or utilization of specific resources) by case-mix category.

Hornbrook's survey[15] offers a way of thinking about case-mix classification, thus providing a conceptual framework for reviewing different methods of constructing clinically meaningful and managerially useful case-mix classifications. In particular, he emphasizes the importance of targeting data to episodes of illness and episodes of care. Lion et al.[16] display a state-of-the-art system, ambulatory visit groups (AVGs), for classifying ambulatory care visits. The AVG system uses information (e.g., patient age, diagnosis, principal procedures) comparable to that employed in the DRG schema for inpatient care. That work, along with that of Rosenblatt et al.[17] on diagnostic clusters for ambulatory care, extends the research on patient classification from the inpatient to the outpatient arena. Rosenblatt et al. discovered that the majority of ambulatory care delivered is represented by a small number (15) of diagnostic clusters.

A relatively untapped opportunity for further work in case-mix classification related to the integration of clinical and financial data lies in the whole area of population-based (e.g., delivery systems offering care on a capitated payment basis) management information systems. Research into integrated data systems has not shown explicitly how to take an episode-based, as compared with visit- or hospitalization-based, approach to defining financial and utilization information for a population. That is essentially the problem HMOs face: attempting to forecast, plan for, and control the utilization and cost-generating experience of a whole population of potential patients. Developing data systems that are population-based, not only for explicitly organized HMOs but also for vertically and horizontally integrated systems of care of other types, clearly will be the next major advance in research and actual practice in the use of integrated systems.

The final set of research on integrated data systems summarized here is oriented toward the development of cost-finding methodologies for case-specific categories of patients. To date, this work has focused exclusively on hospital care and is best represented by a single article in 1982 by Williams et al.[18] As is typical of most studies of case-mix classification and its relationship to cost, that analysis focused on a subset of diagnosis types. The emphasis was on illustrating the difference between cost per DRG identified by two alternate methods:

1. the traditional method, which uses cost-to-charge ratios by departmental cost center, then multiplies those RCCs by the patient's recorded charges to obtain an estimate of cost per patient
2. the direct method, or enumeration of components, which develops standard costs per DRG (more generally, per specific case type) by tracking the actual utilization of materials, labor, and department or cost center-specific overhead for each patient of a given type.

Thus, the research on integrated data systems offers a variety of perspectives— on the one hand, descriptive and cost-accounting focus and, on the other hand, conceptual and empirical, based on consideration of the purposes for integrated data systems, the design of alternate case-mix classification methodologies, and the impact of case-based direct cost accounting.

The next section focuses on interpreting and discussing the results of that research literature in greater detail.

INTEGRATED DATA SYSTEMS

Burik and Duvall[19] present two exhibits directly applicable to the design of cost-accounting systems that integrate clinical and financial information and to the process of developing standard costs for specific case-mix categories. Both exhibits, adapted and summarized here, provide a useful overview of the steps involved in linking clinical and financial data at the level of the individual patient and/or the individual service account.

Figure 9–1 presents a cost-accounting framework for an integrated data system. The diagram is particularly useful in that it summarizes the logical process by which integrated clinical and financial data are developed and displayed.

Figure 9-1 Cost-Accounting Framework for an Integrated Data System

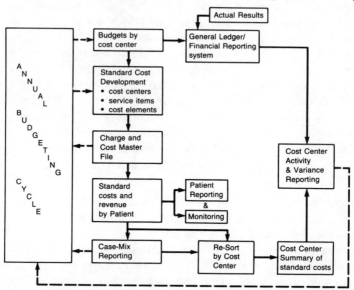

Source: Adapted with permission from the March 1985 issue of *Healthcare Financial Management.*
Copyright 1985, Healthcare Financial Management Association.

The analysis begins with the development of budgets by cost center within the institution or organization. It proceeds to the development of standard costs, first at the level of cost centers, then at the more detailed level of individual service items and broader cost elements. These data flow through to an integrated charge and cost master file that ties together revenue data from patient billing and standard pricing formats with the standard costs developed at the other points in the process.

The data from the charge and cost master file allow the development of standard costs and revenues by individual patients and also feed directly into the annual budgeting cycle. The availability of standard cost and revenue information at the patient level permits the development of case-mix reporting as well as patient-specific reporting and monitoring as a part of the continuing clinical and management functions of the hospital.

Case-Mix and Variance Reporting

Cost centers can resort to case-mix reports to provide a summary of standard costs by important case-mix categories. The cost center summary then flows through to activity and variance reports that address any differences between predicted or budgeted and actual performance. In turn, these activity and variance reports at the cost center level are fed back to the annual budgeting cycle. The process is completed as the budgeting cycle contributes to standard cost development for the next period and provides direct data for constructing the current budget by cost center.

The budgets by cost center provide direct input to the general ledger and financial reporting system for the overall health care organization. Actual results flow directly into the general ledger and financial reporting system, thus providing the basis for continuing analysis of the variances between actual and budgeted performance. The flow diagram of Figure 9–1 essentially recapitulates the logic of an integrated data system and, at the same time, shows the points at which research might contribute most directly to the implementation and improvement of such clinical and financial information systems. For example, the three points at which research might affect such systems most directly are:

1. the development of standard costs and revenue by patient type
2. the design of optimal case-mix classification methods
3. innovation in cost-accounting techniques for reporting variances such as those attributable to volume, mix, price, and efficiency.

Figure 9–2, again summarized and adapted from the same article by Burik and Duvall, outlines in somewhat greater detail the process for developing standard costs. The research contribution here is in providing an integrated linkage between service item-specific standard costing and the specific studies utilized in managing the health care organization. For example, the service item-specific standard costs are particularly useful for pricing the intermediate products of the health services system but also provide valuable input to microcosting (e.g., pricing relative value units for specific procedures within the institution at their marginal cost, input/output costing, analyzing the effects of patient acuity on cost per patient, and developing more specific cost-to-charge ratios).

The development of standard cost, which is advanced considerably by integrating the clinical information on specific patients with the financial system data on cost, is central to the organization's pricing, productivity, service-mix diversification, and goal-setting activities. Thus, in following the logic of Figure 9–2, it becomes clear that the choice of an overall corporate or institutional target or break-even margin on specific kinds of activity will be affected crucially by the organization's ability to meet its standard cost goals for different patient classifications.

A well-formulated and well-monitored standard cost development process is an important element of the integrated data system, with the other major input being provided by a flexible and accurate case-mix classification mechanism.

Figure 9–2 Standard Cost Development Process

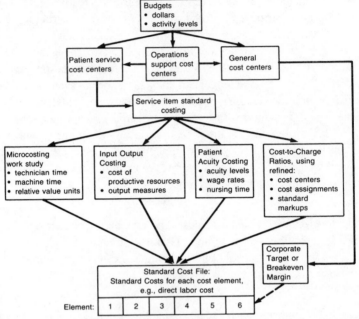

Source: Adapted with permission from the March 1985 issue of *Healthcare Financial Management.* Copyright 1985, Healthcare Financial Management Association.

Framework for an HMO

Bisbee and McCarthy[20] present a conceptual framework and actual reports from a planning, budgeting, and cost control system in use at an operating HMO. The purposes of that system in the HMO are:

- resource allocation
- pricing
- efficiency and cost control
- quality control.

They point out that such integrated data systems in HMOs (as well as in other types of health care institutions) generally have been limited because: (1) administrative and clinical data sets are collected and reported separately and (2) the output of patient care is elusive to define, so the output-based reports of such an integrated data system necessarily are grounded on very general information relating to utilization and financial data. Thus a patient classification scheme over time, as against one that is merely episode specific or visit specific, is a critical component of improved integrated data systems in the HMO context.

Even given these difficulties, the application discussed by Bisbee and McCarthy in the Yale/New Haven Health Plan[2] appears to have succeeded in providing a series of information reports of direct utility to management.

First, a resource consumption profile was developed, which categorized direct/ indirect and total ambulatory cost by diagnostic category. Direct costs were defined as those that varied with and were directly attributable to volume changes, and indirect costs were described as department and total hospital overhead costs. In categorizing the data by diagnosis, the resource consumption profile utilized broad types such as infectious disease, hypertension, and cardiac disease, and diseases of the respiratory tract.

Separately for each of these broad diagnostic categories, financial data were presented on direct costs per visit and in total and on the percentage of direct costs accounted for by each diagnostic category. Similar arrays were displayed for indirect costs and total costs. The planning, budgeting, and cost control system (PBCC) also produced detailed reports within each diagnostic category by all providers, as well as by physician groups and nurse practitioner groups. These analyses provided percentage breakdowns and utilization figures such as the number of visits for laboratory tests and radiological procedures, and the percentage of expenses attributable to nonlaboratory and nonradiological components of ambulatory care.

The data profiles also incorporated information on utilization frequencies of hospital care, intermediate care, and ambulatory care within each diagnostic category, coupled with information on the average cost per visit in each of those factors by diagnostic category.

The reports discussed by Bisbee and McCarthy illustrate that it is practical to develop an integrated data system for an HMO, but it is limited by the highly general definitions of output and means for classifying patients.

Coding Errors and Their Impact

In research descriptive of current integrative data systems in use, Corn[21] reports on errors in coding hospital abstract data and their impact on reimbursement. His discussion is particularly relevant to the development of integrated data systems, all of which rely on some form of diagnostic and patient classification data in order to organize reports. Corn's study says that, on the average, 18.5 percent of all principal diagnostic codes on hospital abstracts were not the same as the codes reconciled retrospectively and 17 percent of all hospital discharges were classified into the wrong DRG. He finds, however, that compensating errors in abstract coding led to a net underpayment of only $8.25 per hospital discharge, a figure not significantly different from zero. He also reports no observable relationship between the net reimbursement error and the individual hospital's error rate in classifying DRGs.

It is interesting to note that Corn's data were drawn from a time (1977) before the use of DRGs for reimbursement in New Jersey. It thus would be important to replicate his study in the current market environment, in which states increasingly are using DRGs for hospital payment. The impact of errors on reimbursement should provide an incentive for accurate coding and a reduction in the frequency of such underlying errors.

THE CONCEPTUAL FRAMEWORK

A second important category of research studies involving integrated data systems addresses the conceptual framework for such systems, the design of case-mix classification mechanisms, and a single rigorous study of the direct method of cost finding at the case-specific level.

Cost-Influencing Variables

A study by Young and Saltman[22] speaks to the importance of isolating cost-influencing variables and matching each of those to the organizational actors or control factors that might affect each of those variables. They describe a set of five key cost-influencing variables: case mix, number of cases treated in the institution, inputs per case (mode of treatment), unit price of inputs, and efficiency of input use. By cross-tabulating each of those variables against a set of four control factors—the environment, physicians, administrators, and third party payers—Young and Saltman conclude that, for control purposes, the variables of case mix and of number of cases will be influenced primarily by the environment. Although case mix and volume are largely beyond the immediate control of physicians, a reporting system still should capture the impact of such variations on cost, revenue, productivity, and profitability at the level of the individual institution.

The Young and Saltman analysis contrasts data system requirements for control purposes with the demands on such systems to provide timely and relevant reporting for planning, budgeting, and retrospective and concurrent analysis purposes. The same analysis relating control factors to cost-influencing variables points out that physicians play the principal role in controlling inputs per case and in determining the mode of treatment. Thus, any integrated data system should direct timely and accurate information to physicians on the utilization of inputs (e.g., ancillary services, length of stay, outside referrals) specific to their practice. Finally, the Young and Saltman analysis implies that input efficiency will be controlled mainly at both the top and middle management levels; thus, data on input use in general and by specific patient classification categories should be targeted to managers and presented in ways that facilitate action.

In sum, Young and Saltman suggest that there is a need to bring together budget formulation and monitoring in a diagnosis-oriented management control system. They also emphasize the need to align controllability and responsibility within the organization by matching cost-influencing variables to the specific control factors that have the primary impact on those variables. The same logic suggests hospital managers should not be held accountable for forces beyond their control. The integrated data system can be viewed as a way of presenting information to specific agents in the institution in ways that permit them to control their functions more effectively.

Variability Control

Griffith's work in cost control for hospitals[23] highlights an important conclusion: where variability exists, it is more effective to control that variability through the scheduling of admissions and control of occupancy than through the development of variable budgets. He emphasizes that for accurate control data, the budget and reporting periods should be the same; the end points of budgeting and reporting periods, respectively, should be the same for each budget grouping; and labor costs must be targeted precisely to the responsibility centers in which they belong and must be tracked frequently by shift within each center.

While Griffith's contribution is not directed specifically to integrated data systems, in the sense of data based on case-mix reporting capability, his observations are important to the design of such systems. The emphasis is on control, rather than variable budgeting, and on accurate assignment of labor costs to each budget grouping. This logic could be extended to suggest that:

1. for an integrated data system, budget and reporting periods within case-mix categories ought to be the same
2. for each diagnostic grouping, the end points of those budgeting and reporting periods ought to be contemporaneous
3. for labor costs (the principal component of total costs), the need is to relate them accurately to responsibility centers within the organization.

To draw a lesson from Young and Saltman, it might be suggested that responsibility centers in an integrated data system would involve programs based on clinically related categories. For example, major diagnostic categories might provide a useful way for the institution to characterize its overall case mix—and for analyzing its labor costs by the major components of its service mix.

Integrated Records

Steinwachs's research[24] speaks directly to future developments for ambulatory care management information systems. However, the general structure of the integrated data system he discusses is transferable to inpatient care and, more generally, to population-based systems. He discusses three types of records, each of which must be merged and integrated for a comprehensive data system to fulfill its purposes:

1. A patient registration record that incorporates:

   - a unique patient identifier
   - patient name
   - address
   - source(s) of payment
   - birthdate
   - sex

2. A provider identification record that includes:

   - a unique provider identifier
   - provider name
   - specialty of provider
   - location of the provider's practice

3. A visits, or encounter, record that includes:

   - date
   - place of service
   - type of visit
   - patient I.D.
   - provider I.D.
   - diagnostic services
   - diagnosis or problem
   - therapeutic services delivered at the encounter
   - preventive services delivered
   - status upon disposition (e.g., discharged to hospital, referred to another specialty provider)
   - total charges.

Steinwachs emphasizes that the primary purposes of such an integrated data system are to provide timely and influential information on provider productivity and on the appropriateness of utilization and the outcomes of care.

The Feedback Factor

He identifies the potential for a more effective role of management information systems in providing feedback to managers concerning problem areas and potential opportunities and to providers concerning diagnostic or treatment options or deficiencies in the quality of care. This kind of emphasis on clinical feedback can provide a useful complement to the historical emphasis on applications to support management decision making.

As Steinwachs and others have recognized, however, feedback strategies have their own limitations, and the use of integrated data systems for feedback purposes should take these into account. As he points out, the threshold for identifying problem areas must be identified uniquely in each setting. The costs and benefits of initiating action depend on the institution's environment, mix of reimbursement sources, corresponding differences in the reimbursement methods of third party payers, and organizational structure. Thus, in setting up criteria for using management information system outputs to identify problems, an institution-by-institution analysis is necessary.

He also says there seems to be little agreement concerning which problem areas should be the target of information systems feedback. He observes that the information provided by financial management information systems is strong in identifying historical patterns, such as overdue accounts receivable and other indexes of financial liability, but considerably weaker in offering timely information for devising sophisticated cash management strategies. Finally, and more important, the development of feedback strategies can proceed effectively only to the extent that criteria for the appropriate and efficient practice of medicine are defined clearly and consensually.

The essence of feedback strategies resulting from integrated data relies on communication with and involvement of physicians. Until agreed and operational criteria are established for specific areas of medical practice, such feedback mechanisms will have limited effect on utilization patterns and physician practices. State-of-the-art data systems are not enough; criteria for action and standards for medical and administrative practice are necessary preconditions for data to generate efficient and effective managerial and clinical behavior.

IMPACT AND ROLE OF DRGs

Conceptual issues in the design of case-mix classification techniques comprise an important theme of research contributing to the development of integrated data systems. The use of DRGs in the Medicare prospective pricing system (PPS) has led to major focus on DRGs as a patient classification method; the literature on case-mix classification reflects this. However, for the management and clinical teams designing an integrated data system, the patient classification mechanism should not be taken as a given but rather as an element of choice based on the purposes for which the data will be employed.

Research by Horn and Schumacher[25] concentrates on explaining variation in charges and length of stay within DRG categories, using as an example acute myocardial infarction (AMI). They use two new categorization concepts for patient mix: the physician data optimal system (MD-DATO) and a patient severity system they developed.

The MD-DATO system is derived primarily from considerations of medical meaningfulness and charge homogeneity within (for example) the AMI category. It takes into account the secondary diagnoses most likely to explain differences in charges and mortality rates among acute myocardial infarction patients. The AS-SCORE categorization technique, which is an index of inpatient severity of illness, simultaneously reflects the patient's age, stage of disease, complications, and response to therapy.

In regard to the data on charges for AMI patients, the MD-DATO classification reduced variance by 4 to 5 percent within DRG categories, the AS-SCORE technique by 14 percent. Results were similar in a large metropolitan medical center teaching hospital and a 300-bed community hospital with no teaching programs. The improved classification (as measured by the reduction in variance in charges within the DRG category) was not statistically significant in the teaching medical center but was in the community hospital.

In contrast, the AS-SCORE index achieved further improvement in classification in relation to the DRG category for both the teaching medical center and the community hospital. Both the physician data optimal system and the patient severity index significantly improved classification relative to the DRG in terms of length of stay in a community hospital. However, neither significantly reduced variances in relation to DRGs in the teaching medical center. In general, the data suggest that incremental classification beyond DRG categories does create more homogeneous case-mix classifications.

COST OF CREATING CATEGORIES

The question for management and for an integrated data system is the cost of creating these incremental categories, and the benefits to management and to clinical practice of doing so. As of early 1986, the research had not addressed the question of the cost effectiveness of alternative case-mix classification schemes. Nor was there a consensus on whether this classification should focus exclusively on the patient's presenting conditions at time of entry to the health care system or should also take into account how that particular set of conditions was treated and the trajectory of responses to therapy. An important question for data system use and adoption is the extent to which such systems are meant to classify presenting problems versus classifying not only presenting problems but also the system's response to those problems.

The work of Gonnella[26] stresses the importance of considering disease processes as dynamic, not static, and for reducing the heterogeneity within alternative patient-mix categories. The philosophy of the team of investigators with whom Gonnella has worked[27] in developing a disease staging case-mix classification incorporates information on the categories and etiological agents contributing to the disease, the stage of the disease itself, and the organ system involved. They emphasize that the case-mix classification should not include the nature of the medical intervention for a particular patient in the initial separation of case-mix groupings within the classification.

Thus, the use of the disease staging approach to case-mix classification would focus on the presenting problem and would not classify a given case according to how it was treated. Management has an important choice to make here: Does it desire a classification scheme that simultaneously measures the presenting problem and how it was treated, or does it want to obtain as homogeneous a measure as possible of the presenting problem and relate that to cost, charges, length of stay, and other data demonstrating how that problem was treated in the health care institution or system?

Management's choice in the context of an integrated data system turns on the uses to which that information will be applied. If a system's primary purpose is to achieve control and monitoring of practice patterns, then the classifying system should not include details on how a presenting problem was treated but rather should focus on identifying the problem's homogeneous categories.

Hornbrook[28] repeats the view of Gonnella that case-mix classifications should be derived according to clinically relevant characteristics of the patient, in that the measure should include no utilization or treatment choice factors. His logic for that preference is instructive, as he points out that inclusion of the utilization factor has two possible impacts: (1) it may build in an implicit assumption that treatment or utilization was appropriate and (2) its use of utilization factors in case-mix classification may lead to incentives to shift the classification in directions that increase reimbursement and/or make providers look better on certain internal screens for clinical and managerial performance.

Hornbrook points out that the actual choice of treatment regimen may depend more on the structure of physician fees and other economic and social determinants of the rewards of performing different procedures than on the hospital reimbursement rate for specific DRGs or patient-mix categories. If this is correct, and the author tends to agree, then the integrated data system seeking to analyze provider behavior and practice patterns must take into account such factors external to the hospital.

For example, the data system needs to be rich enough to incorporate information on physician fees and the medical malpractice premium consequences of alternative treatment choices so that the impact of these factors on clinical decision making can be factored into the analysis of utilization patterns at the institution. Such factors may be taken into account simply by developing simulation models in the integrated data system that can project the impact on hospital revenues and costs of alternative physician fee and hospital payment structures for specific procedures and types of service.

AMBULATORY VISIT GROUPS

An important empirical contribution by Lion et al.[29] involves utilization of ambulatory visit groups (AVGs) in a prospective payment system for outpatient care. AVGs, first developed by Fetter,[30] classify visits into 14 major diagnostic groups, based on organ system. A series of clustering variables is included in the AVG algorithm to reduce the variance in physician time per visit within each AVG. Those clustering variables include presenting problem, reason for visit, primary diagnosis, presence or absence of a secondary diagnosis, visit types, and patient age. Coupled with the finding by Rosenblatt et al.,[31] that some 50 percent of ambulatory care can be accounted for by as few as 15 diagnostic clusters, the potential applicability of AVGs for classifying ambulatory care visits is striking.

A series of management information reports could be generated from a system using AVGs as the ambulatory classification tool involving:

- cost per visit by AVG
- characterization of patient mix using a frequency distribution of the most common AVGs for internists, general practitioners, and physician subspecialties related to primary care
- comparison of physician time input and physician assistant/nursing time input for the most common AVGs with the standard in the AVG classification system
- analysis of the range of physician and other personnel time input per visit within common AVGs, such as identifying the time variability by examining the high and the low time or by comparing profiles for different providers
- comparison of current pricing patterns by type of visit (AVG) and mean time input.

This kind of management report would characterize the case-mix of the ambulatory patients and provide administration with useful information as to how the treatment team is responding to that patient stream.

One of the inferences drawn by Lion's study team was that an episode-of-illness approach might be intuitively attractive but would involve certain difficulties (although not necessarily intractable ones). Particularly for chronic conditions requiring ambulatory care, the identification of a beginning and end of the episode would be difficult. Perhaps for management purposes, it is enough to know the primary nature of the presenting problem and to stratify patient visits over time into the primary reason for the visit. However, moving to an episode-of-illness approach would indeed be difficult for such cases.

The system as a whole means all individual health care institutions seeking to track their patients' utilization of services outside a particular facility, in the sense of the community of institutions in a given market. One means by which that system as a whole might respond to the difficulties in defining the case type for chronic illnesses would be to leapfrog the question of episodes and focus on a fixed interval of time as the unit of analysis. Essentially, this is what HMOs do. The issue then becomes one of categorizing patients as to their primary health problems prevailing over time, as against categorizing individual visits, admissions, or even episodes.

Steinwachs[32] does suggest a type of episode-based analysis that might be useful for more acute problems. It would focus on measurement of the duration of the episode, mix of services utilized, the presence and identity of single and/or multiple providers, and the total cost of the episode. Useful information for management would include reports of the alternative patterns of care and total cost of treatment within episodes under the direction of a primary care physician, as against those treated by a nurse practitioner or a physician's assistant. This episode-based approach would provide a means for examining differences over time in treatment patterns and cost consequences for alternative categories of health care provider.

DIRECT COST FINDING VS. RCC

The literature makes clear that there is a need for further research on case-mix measures in relation to populations served on a capitation payment basis and on the development of case-mix measures related to episodes of illness. In addition, any episode-based information system would have to confront the fundamental problem of reliably linking services into unique episodes of illness. Perhaps as a compromise strategy, the analyst and management might end up dealing with episodes of care, as against episodes of illness, in the initial classification.

The final theme in the literature on integrated data systems is represented in the 1982 analysis by Williams and colleagues,[33] who compare two cost-finding methodologies for case-specific hospitalization episodes. They contrast a direct cost-finding method and a more traditional (RCC) approach. Their study is rich in implications for integrated data systems, for they provide the first published information on the difference in cost measurements derived from RCC methods as against a more direct tracking of variable and fixed expenses by patient. Hence, their work indirectly offers guidance on whether the information system should be built upon more detailed transaction-specific information at the level of the individual episode or on broad averages of the type used in the RCC methodology, which implicitly assumes that the cost-to-charge ratio is constant across service items within a given cost center.

The Williams study, which compared the two cost methodologies for DRG 198 and DRG 199 (inguinal hernia repair without obstruction, with and without major secondary diagnosis, respectively) found that the measured total costs per DRG under the direct approach were approximately two-thirds of those when using the traditional RCC method. Those proportionate differences held up for both DRGs. The direction of these differences was maintained in each of the specific cost centers on which the study team concentrated (operating room, radiology, and clinical laboratory), although the differences were most pronounced for operating room cost.

For example, measured operating room cost per hospitalization under the direct method was $118.06 for DRG 199 as compared with $204.01 for the same DRG under the traditional cost-finding method. Williams et al. did not examine general hospital overhead, e.g., administration, building depreciation, and interest, but chose instead to focus on cost centers involving activity that was likely to vary with respect to treatment volumes and the underlying condition being treated.

An important question for future research, given the differences observed in that study, would be the impact of using a direct vs. a traditional method for a costlier DRG (in which the direction of the findings might be reversed, with the direct methodology likely to uncover greater costs than the overall average implicitly utilized by the RCC approach).

A second important research question concerns the cost effectiveness of obtaining more accurate information at the individual patient level, given that the direct tracking of time and resources utilized per patient implies greater cost of collecting information. Such information requires certain manual time-and-motion studies and other data inputs that, while they can be incorporated into an integrated data system, do imply greater informational requirements and a decision as to how often to update the detailed information and assumptions.

VALUE OF THE RESEARCH

To return to an element in the earlier taxonomy on integrated data systems, specifically that concerned with the adoption vs. the utilization of this "new technology," the research does appear to provide good descriptions of current systems in use and the reporting capabilities they provide. The literature is replete with details on alternative case-mix classification schemes, which are an important part of an integrated data system and which provide important keys to how that system will be used in a given institution or other setting. The research appears to be less useful generally in answering the question as to which kind of integrated system a given hospital should adopt.

Details on the relevant software and hardware for integrated data systems are only beginning to emerge in the literature.

A 1985 article as part of the series by Burik and Duvall[34] exemplifies this literature in its presentation of a list of hospital cost management systems software vendors. Those authors do not pretend that their list is all-inclusive, pointing out the rapid marketplace evolution of software. The principal variation in costing software, which is just one part of an integrated data system (although the major component stressed in the literature), is in the capacity for developing standard costs presented by each software package.

Thus, perhaps the key element for decision making in adopting hospital costing software is management's desire to develop fine-tuned cost measurements by patient, by service, and by charge item, and for variance reporting. As Burik and Duvall report, most vendors have designed flexible software for writing reports documenting a variance between actual and budgeted or predicted performance. The evolution of integrated data systems therefore will turn significantly on the capacities of individual institutions to generate the information they need for specific reports.

Nathanson[35] summarizes the state-of-the-art as of 1983 by suggesting that then-available computerized data systems gave strong representation of the macro picture confronting health care institutions but did not appear to include enough details on which administrators and physicians and other health care providers could act. An important constraint on the extent of future innovation in data systems technology is the need for clinical norms for the utilization of ancillary services, length of stay, physician input, and nursing effort per patient-mix category (e.g., DRGs). In addition, the adoption and use of integrated data systems in small hospitals may be hampered by the absence of sufficient cases per type.

Logically, this suggests that, for innovation, smaller institutions might use a different and perhaps more aggregated patient-mix classification as compared with those of larger hospitals. The pressure for linking data on financial and clinical behavior in a market environment of prospective payment by case-mix classification categories will encourage smaller institutions to form systems not only for the delivery of care but also for the analysis of data.

Nathanson discusses the use of DRGs as possible accounting categories and notes that, as Simborg has pointed out,[36] DRGs are "soft" categories for cost finding. In this respect, the adoption and use of clinical feedback systems pose both the greatest challenge and the greatest potential growth area in cost-containment software in the coming years.

Another factor is analysis of the contributions of research in the areas of reporting, planning, budgeting, and controlling health care institutional and system performance. As the author perceives it, the general thrust of the literature has been particularly useful in suggesting means for reporting historical and current data in more productive ways; for example, by targeting differing physician profiles by DRG and by isolating costs by DRG within a cost center in the facility that vary markedly from the institutional averages provided by the information systems.

The integrated data system also will have clear-cut application to planning the service mix in the future, especially as case-mix-specific reports on profitability, cost, and revenue patterns are presented. Inevitably, the integrated management information system will be able to isolate the impact of alternative clinical treatment regimens and patient-mix categories on the financial health of the institution and to display a description of its current portfolio of activities. Both purposes are important—not only the evaluation of performance but also the description in a strategic planning sense of the current operating portfolio.

Burik and Duvall[37] also outline how hospitals might use effectively an integrated data system to present their product line profit and loss statements, i.e., income statements specific to particular DRGs or other product line/patient-mix classification categories.

The application of the outputs of integrated data systems for planning product pricing strategies is likely to be demonstrated convincingly in the short term. Burik and Duvall conclude that even small hospitals should not substitute an RCC approach for more detailed direct cost finding in determining service item-specific standard costs. They argue that, on the cost side, such figures are too highly aggregated within each department; on the charge side, they again are too highly aggregated and thus obscure the impact of changing product mix and different price markups among the service items in a department. In summary, the relevance of integrated data system outputs for reporting and product pricing and planning purposes appears to be immediate and direct.

In contrast, the research does not necessarily demonstrate the effectiveness of integrated data system outputs for budgeting and controlling functions. It also does not show the practicability of developing a case-mix-specific budgeting system. Indeed, to the extent that there are small numbers of cases in a significant number of the case types (e.g., DRGs), budgeting on a case-specific basis would be difficult and possibly unreliable at the level of the individual cost center or major diagnostic category.

However, it appears likely that effective control strategies can be developed by case-specific reports—for example, physician-specific and DRG-specific profiles of cost, revenue, and utilization of services and resources. This is an area with particularly great potential for a case-based integrated data system. As Young and Saltman argue,[38] the advantage of case-based analysis and reporting is that it clarifies the impact of differing modes of treatment (such as input use patterns) on the cost of health services.

An integrated data system with case-specific reporting capacity thus provides management and clinicians with a unique tool for identifying variances from standard practice. The key advance that must be made to realize this potential, however, is the further evolution in standards and norms of practice for efficient and effective input use by specific case-mix categories. Until that happens, the impact of integrated data systems on the control function in health care institutions will be limited.

AGENDA FOR FUTURE RESEARCH

These comments on the value of previous research on integrated data systems for reporting, planning, budgeting, and controlling in health care suggest an important agenda for future research. Much of this amounts to joining previously disparate streams of empirical and theoretical inquiry. The kinds of questions to be confronted are comprehensive in nature and demand integration of clinical and financial research pathways that previously have been largely separate.

This analysis has highlighted several themes on work that needs to be done. This section pulls those themes together into a coherent whole.

Cost-Effective Alternatives

First, the field of health administration practice needs to get a handle on which among the alternative approaches to integrated data systems is the most cost effective for each of the four major purposes. The questions of what kind of information systems capacity to build, which particular software packages to utilize, and which mechanisms for patient classification to use all are intimately related and are important in evaluating the utility of a particular system.

Careful research is needed on the trade-offs in collecting more detailed (through direct cost-finding methods) input data and the benefits accruing from such information. The research should articulate the difference between (1) the data system's contribution to reporting historical performance and strategic planning for the institution's future service mix portfolio and (2) the real-time application of such integrated data system reports for program and institutional budgeting and the control of cost center and individual clinician/manager performance.

The example of direct cost-finding vs. traditional cost-finding (RCC) raises a classic question: Is the apparent greater precision provided by the direct method worth the incremental cost of collecting such data? In addressing such a question, research is needed on the cost to the institution of collecting more detailed information (conducting the underlying time-and-motion and other special studies), and the consequent changes in behavior resulting from the provision of more accurate information.

It seems clear that in a competitive marketplace the benefits of DRG and other case-specific information on cost will be instrumental in designing more effective pricing structures. However, the research should document behavior change in physicians, managers, patients, and so on, as a function of the provision of information. This can illustrate whether or not detailed case-based data have resulted in budgeting and control that correspond to the somewhat clearer advantages of integrated data system information for retrospective reporting and broad-based strategic planning and pricing.

Merger of the Data Files

Second, another important stream of research would address a practical issue: the finding in the Burik and Duvall study that a significant technical problem with integrated data systems was the merger of the clinical and financial data files. Specifically, the matching algorithm used in the system they discussed was unable to link the correct bill consistently with the correct abstract in a particular application.

Research is needed on a variety of distinct integrated data systems, outlining the practical problems concerning that linkage of clinical and financial data files. What appears as a simple point of linking patient identification numbers or patient names, birthdates, and other verifying individual level information often turns out in practice to be a much more complicated matter. The field needs a kind of inventory of these difficulties and a sense of the priority of their importance and degree of tractability.

In the same vein of data linkage, it is clear that methods have not been developed sufficiently for reliably linking services and episodes. If episode-based and person-based systems of presenting information are to represent the next generation of data systems, research is needed on a definition of episodes that will facilitate the linking of particular health care services at specific times to a given episode of illness.

Population-Based Systems

These episode-of-illness questions lead into the next higher level of aggregation—that is, an integrated, population-based system of the type required for an HMO. For this development, new ways are needed for categorizing the population beyond age, sex, and socioeconomic indicators. Those kinds of population attributes will be a necessary adjunct to characterizing patients' health characteristics over the long term or to defining the clinical and psychosocial problem presented by a patient to the broader health care system over a given period.

The literature reports the development of a variety of patient classification methodologies attuned to characterizing the ambulatory care visit or the episode of hospitalization; the next generation for research and implementation is to derive similar classification schema for patients over time, or at least within episodes of illness. Such patient-classification or, more accurately, person-classification methods, designed for the health care system's planning and performance evaluation, will be increasingly vital to the development of intelligent integrated data systems. Clinical and financial data for a continuing system cannot be integrated without a means of characterizing the patient over time vs. over a single transaction or episode.

On this same theme of population-based data systems, it is clear that research is needed into the feasibility and characteristics of a vertically integrated patient record—that is, an integrated record over time for the individual that correlates clinical conditions and characteristics of care providers with the financial data summarizing that patient's transactions with the health care system. To do that, research should look at how best to link outpatient and inpatient records across a variety of providers in the health care system for a given individual.

The technical issues concern data linkage on some common patient identifier across a variety of organizationally distinct health care units, the definition of a uniform abstract for financial data (perhaps modeled along the lines of the UB82 developed by the Health Care Financing Administration), and the reconciliation of potentially different definitions for health care outputs (e.g., the coding of an individual ambulatory care visit as of limited, intermediate, or long duration).

Increasingly, as the field moves to integrate clinical and financial data, it will encounter the "softness" of patient classification categories such as DRGs when used as cost-accounting categories. Both researchers and practitioners in administration and delivery of care will need to develop and evaluate new means of clinically classifying patients and populations that also are economically meaningful in identifying cost and revenue streams. Indeed, this is crucial, for if integrated data systems are to realize their promise, they must contribute to improved clinical performance as well as management practice.

NOTES

1. D. Burik and T.J. Duvall, "Hospital Cost Accounting: Strategic Considerations," *Health Care Financial Management* 15, no. 2 (1985): 19–28.

2. G.E. Bisbee, Jr., and M.M. McCarthy, "Planning, Budgeting, and Cost Control in HMOs," in *Managing the Finances of Health Care Organizations,* ed. G.E. Bisbee, Jr., and R. Vraciu (Ann Arbor: Health Administration Press, 1980): 202.

3. Richard F. Corn, "The Sensitivity of Prospective Hospital Reimbursement to Errors in Patient Data," *Inquiry* 18, no. 1 (1981): 351–60.

4. D. Burik and T.J. Duvall, "Hospital Cost Accounting: Finding the Software Solution," *Health Care Financial Management* 15, no. 4 (1985): 76–84.

5. _____, "Hospital Cost Accounting: Implementing the System Successfully," *Health Care Financial Management* 15, no. 15 (1985): 76–88.

6. Bisbee and McCarthy, "Planning, Budgeting," 19–28.

7. Corn, "Sensitivity," 351–60.

8. J. Lion et al., "Ambulatory Visit Groups: A Prospective Payment System for Outpatient Care," *Journal of Ambulatory Care Management* 7, no. 4 (1984): 30–45.

9. R.A. Rosenblatt et al., "The Content of Ambulatory Care in the United States: An Interspecialty Comparison," *New England Journal of Medicine* 309 (1983): 892–97.

10. D.W. Young and R.B. Saltman, "Preventive Medicine for Hospital Costs," *Harvard Business Review* 83, no. 1 (1983): 126–33.

11. J.R. Griffith, "Criteria and Procedures for Establishing Accounting Based Control Systems," in *Cost Control in Hospitals,* ed. J.R. Griffith et al. (Ann Arbor, Mich.: Health Administration Press, 1976), 269.

12. D.M. Steinwachs, "Ambulatory Care Management Information Systems: Future Directions," *Journal of Ambulatory Care Management* 8, no. 2 (1985): 84–94.

13. S.D. Horn and D.N. Schumacher, "Comparing Classification Methods: Measurement of Variations in Charges, Length of Stay, and Mortality," *Medical Care* 20, no. 5 (1982): 489–500.

14. J.S. Gonnella, "Patient Case Mix: Implications for Medical Education and Hospital Costs," *Journal of Medical Education* 56 (1981): 610–11.

15. M.C. Hornbrook, "Hospital Case Mix: Its Definition, Measurement and Use: Part II. Review of Alternative Measures," *Medical Care Review* 39, no. 2 (1982): 73–123.

16. Lion et al., "Ambulatory Visit Groups," 30–45.

17. Rosenblatt et al. "Content of Ambulatory Care," 892–97.

18. Sankey V. Williams et al., "Improved Cost Allocation in Case-Mix Accounting," *Medical Care* 20, no. 5 (1982): 450–59.

19. D. Burik and T.J. Duvall, "Hospital Cost Accounting: A Basic System Framework," *Health Care Financial Management* 15, no. 3 (1985): 58–64.

20. Bisbee and McCarthy, "Planning, Budgeting," 202.

21. Corn, "Sensitivity," 351–60.

22. Young and Saltman, "Preventive Medicine," 126–33.

23. Griffith, "Criteria and Procedures."

24. Steinwachs, "Ambulatory Care," 84–94.

25. Horn and Schumacher, "Comparing Classification Methods," 489–500.

26. Gonnella, "Patient Case Mix."

27. M.L. Garg et al., "Evaluating Inpatient Costs: The Staging Mechanism," 16 (1981): 191–201.

28. Hornbrook, "Hospital Case Mix," 73–123.

29. Lion et al., "Ambulatory Visit Groups," 892–97.

30. R.B. Fetter, "Ambulatory Patient-Related Groups." (Unpublished manuscript, 1980).

31. Rosenblatt et al., "Content of Ambulatory Care."

32. Steinwachs, "Ambulatory Care," 84–94.

33. Williams et al., "Improved Cost Allocation," 450–59.

34. Burik and Duvall, "Hospital Cost Accounting: Finding the Software Solution," 76–84.

35. M.N. Nathanson, "Computers Crank Out DRG Cost Data, But How Valid is the Information?" *Modern Healthcare* 13, no. 9 (1983): 160–64.

36. Donald M. Simborg, noted in Nathanson, "Computers Crank Out DRG Cost Data," 160.

37. Burik and Duvall, "Hospital Cost Accounting: Implementing the System Successfully," 76–88.

38. Young and Saltman, "Preventive Medicine."

Chapter 10

A Nursing Information System: Needs and Benefits

Kathleen T. Lucke, Linda J. Porter-Stubbs,
Marilyn L. Price, and *Anna Ferguson*

To those who have followed the escalating costs of health care since the mid-1960s, the mandated cost-containment efforts of the 1980s came as no surprise and, in fact, were overdue. The challenge of controlling health care costs while maintaining the right of quality service for all individuals is difficult, with implications extending into many facets of society. To accomplish this goal, health care providers must leave their altruism behind and learn to identify and balance the potential benefits of the many aspects of client care with the costs of providing those services, while delivering an increasingly consumer-defined product.

This, then, is nursing's challenge: to clearly define and accept accountability for the product offered—professional nursing. To respond effectively to this challenge, it is necessary to explore the factors that have contributed to soaring health care costs as well as to understand the implications of the resulting legislation.

In 1966, Titles 18 and 19 of the Social Security Act (P.L. 89-97) established Medicare and Medicaid, perhaps in part in response to the human rights movements of the 1960s. This began an evolving change in the financial structure of the nation's health care system with significant, long-range implications. From 1960 to 1980, the cost for most goods and services increased dramatically while health care costs soared disproportionately and by 1982 were increasing at three times the national inflation rate. In 1965, health care services consumed 5.9 percent of the gross national product (GNP) and, by 1982, 10.5 percent. Consumer prices jumped 250 percent over that period while health care costs soared 550 percent. From 1978 to 1982, Medicare costs rose at an average annual rate of 19 percent— and American taxpayers pay for 40 percent of all hospital bills through Medicare and Medicaid.[1] These figures leave little doubt that health care service needs must be evaluated closely before the system reaches an unsupportable level, as has been suggested by the predictions that Social Security will be bankrupt as early as the 1990s.

CAUSES OF HIGH HEALTH CARE COSTS

To respond effectively to the challenge of providing cost-efficient, quality health care for all individuals, it is necessary first to explore the factors that have contributed to the soaring costs. These factors fall into several major areas:

- The number of persons over age 65 who qualify for and use Social Security benefits is increasing nationally, and they are living longer. Meanwhile, the number of persons contributing to the support of these services is decreasing.
- The nation historically has poor health habits and its health services have focused on treatment and cure rather than prevention. There is an ever-increasing number of persons with chronic illnesses such as heart disease, hypertension, diabetes, chronic obstructive pulmonary disease (COPD), and substance abuse. The long-term repetitive treatment and follow-through needed for these persons have increased health care expenditures significantly.
- Inflation has affected health care expenditures because it has increased costs to providers for equipment, supplies, personnel, etc.
- There was little incentive (before the advent of prospective payment in 1982) for either providers or consumers to be cost effective because of the presence of third party payers and coverage through Social Security.
- The retrospective reimbursement system encouraged increased spending. To make money, health care providers had to spend money. Therefore, the development or expansion of services was encouraged for their financial benefits.
- Uninformed individuals historically have been the passive recipients of health care instead of being actively involved, discriminating, decision-making consumers.

Each of these factors individually could have a potentially negative effect on health care costs; however, in combination, they produced the dangerous spiralling of costs with which the nation now must contend. To contain costs effectively it is necessary to deal with each of these factors individually while recognizing their synergistic and sometimes symbiotic relationships.

The changing demographics and the economic state of the nation are beyond the direct control or influence of health care providers, but the other factors are not. Preventive health care is gaining wider acceptance and a greater following that could be facilitated by community awareness and education. Active consumerism is being accepted and encouraged as public knowledge increases and legislative supports are developed.

Third party payers as well as federally funded programs are evaluating services more closely and expecting consumers to be increasingly responsible financially for their own health care. They are decreasing the percentage of coverage allowed, limiting the types of services provided, rewarding clients who practice preventive health care by reducing their costs, and leaving the higher costs to those clients most at risk for problems. Third party payers are contracting with specific health care providers in exclusive agreements and are reimbursing only for those services. The retrospective reimbursement system under Medicare and Medicaid was replaced with a prospective payment system (PPS). To identify fully what is occurring in health care, and the potential impact of these changes, it is necessary to review the legislative history that brought it about.

LEGISLATIVE HISTORY

As noted earlier, Titles 18 and 19 of the Social Security Act established Medicare and Medicaid in 1966 in response to the desire to provide health care to all members of society. Health care became a right for all Americans, not merely a privilege for those who could afford it. Services were expanded to incorporate the entire population and costs began to rise. By 1972, they had been identified as a major national problem and Section 223 of the Social Security Act was amended to give the Secretary of the then Department of Health, Education, and Welfare (changed to Health and Human Services in 1979) the authority to set limits on routine health care costs. This was part of the Economic Stabilization Program of 1971–1974 and did slow the rate of increases, but not sufficiently.

By 1977 the soaring costs led to the establishment of the Voluntary Effort Program. This was designed to encourage voluntary cost containment by health care providers. It, too, proved ineffective. President Carter tried to make this program mandatory, but intensive lobbying efforts by the health care industry blocked the attempt. In 1982, the Tax Equity and Fiscal Responsibility Act (TEFRA) (P.L. 97-248) was enacted. It added all other costs to Section 223 of the Social Security Act (e.g., education, malpractice, etc.). In 1983, the Social Security Amendments (P.L. 98-21) mandated that Medicare switch to prospective payment based on 467 diagnosis related groups (DRGs). In essence, these bills also set the scene for potential similar action for all health care services in the future.

PROSPECTIVE REIMBURSEMENT/DRGs

Table 10–1 defines the major components of and differences between prospective and retrospective reimbursement.The mechanism chosen for classifying patients for prospective reimbursement is diagnosis related groups, or DRGs. This

Table 10–1 Retrospective vs. Prospective Reimbursement

Retrospective Reimbursement: Cost-Based	Prospective Reimbursement: Case-Based
• Pays all costs from an itemized bill (may include a built-in profit margin); cost of care thus is established after services are provided and patient is discharged.	• Sets rates before care is given based on: location and type of hospital, the hospital's case-mix index, national geometric mean costs, and patient's assigned DRG.
• Tends to be inflationary; to make a dollar, a dollar must be spent.	• Tends not to be inflationary; to make a dollar, a dollar must be saved.
• Encourages increased services, treatments, and longer, more frequent hospitalizations.	• Encourages cost-efficient health care services, with shorter and less frequent hospitalizations.

process was developed through a grant by Yale University using the ICD-9-CM (International Classification of Diseases, 9th edition, Clinical Modification Revision). Twenty-three major diagnostic categories, or MDCs, were identified. These were further broken down into 467 DRGs according to secondary diagnosis, sex, age, surgical procedure, discharge status, and complications. This breakdown allowed for some of the many individual differences between patients with the same major medical diagnoses. The following is an example of this breakdown:

MDC 5: Diseases and Disorders of the Circulatory System:
DRG 103: Heart Transplant
105: Cardiac Valve Procedure with Pump (with and without catheterization)
107: Coronary Bypass (with and without catheterization)
122: Circulatory Disorders with Acute Myocardial Infarction (with and without cardiovascular complications), discharged alive
123: Circulatory Disorder with Acute Myocardial Infarction, expired
130: Peripheral Vascular Disorders age < 69 and/or secondary diagnosis
131: Peripheral Vascular Disorders age 70 without secondary diagnosis

The national geometric mean costs for each DRG were established by evaluating groups of cases for cost-of-stay (COS) and length-of-stay (LOS) data. The sample number differs greatly among DRGs so the geometric mean cost within each DRG may not be representative of the entire patient population. A standard deviation of 1.97 from the mean was identified to allow for a range of "normal" patients for whom the mean established cost of reimbursement would be appropriate. Patients falling outside either (or both) the COS or LOS range of normal are identified as outliers; it was expected that they would represent 4 to 5 percent of the patient population.

Individual patient DRG assignments are made after the individual is discharged by reviewing documentation on the principle diagnosis, secondary diagnosis, age, sex, any surgical procedures performed, complications, and discharge status. The health care provider's reimbursement for the patient is based on the assigned DRG's prospective reimbursement rate for that institution, including preestablished standardized adjustment for the type and location of the institution, its case mix, and any pass-through moneys for education, malpractice, acuity, etc., that it receives. Thus, an institution may make a profit or lose money, depending upon whether or not it can contain its costs within this preestablished limit. Institutions may appeal for additional reimbursement for their outlier population, but they will be asked to justify the additional costs or length of hospitalization.

REVIEW PROCESS

The law established a review process to assure compliance with the prospective payment system (PPS) and DRG assignments. Each state may adopt its own legislation to facilitate this review process or the federal government may identify an existing system to act on its behalf. The components of the review include:

- Five percent of all cases, or every 20th case, will be reviewed.
- Admissions will be evaluated for medical necessity and appropriateness.
- Patient care will be evaluated to ensure similar quality for all patients.
- All interfacility transfers will be reviewed for medical appropriateness.
- Readmissions for the same or related problems will be reviewed.
- All admissions within seven days of discharge from any acute care facility will be reviewed.
- All outliers will be reviewed for reimbursement purposes.
- All fatalities will be reviewed (to determine whether there were excesses or deficiencies).
- All pacemaker implants will be reviewed.

This process will help the federal government identify compliance problems but does not assist the institution involved in identifying problems inherent in the system. Thus, institutions must be aware of, and active in, identifying these system problems.

INSTITUTIONAL PROBLEMS AND CONCERNS

Several aspects of the prospective payment system may prove to be problems, and institutions should be actively involved in evaluating them. The first of these is the institution's designated case-mix index, which is intended to represent the expected classification types and volumes of patients served. The case-mix index upon which reimbursement is established was based on data obtained through a historic review of patients' admission information. Because principle diagnoses frequently are not identified at admission, the case-mix index may not be accurate when compared with that obtained by reviewing discharge information.

Thus, it may be beneficial for institutions to review their discharge data internally and validate their case-mix index, appealing for reimbursement changes as necessary. They also should review supply and wage information periodically to identify significant changes that might affect their reimbursement status. They also should communicate with other similar institutions concerning their case-mix indexes and geometric mean costs.

A second concern with PPS is the potential for shifts in services among institutions to compete for those that are profitable. As institutions gather data on which of their services are and are not profitable, they may opt to make changes that decrease their potential for financial losses. This "dumping" of nonprofitable patients or services will make it more difficult for some persons to obtain specific types of care and will place a financial drain on the public general hospitals left to bear the increasing burden of nonprofitable services. This may push the nation closer to a society with various levels of health care that depend upon ability to pay and back toward a point where health care no longer is a right but a privilege.

The PPS does not account adequately for varying degrees of patient acuity within each DRG. Research determining such patient acuity ranges, based on severity of illness and nursing intensity, is necessary to identify the true resource consumption of individual patients. Such data would be useful in establishing a more accurate reimbursement mechanism as well as in appealing outlier cases.

Another concern with PPS is the cutoff or trim points used to establish outlier status. New Jersey found, upon implementing this system, that 30 percent of its patients fell into the outlier category instead of the 4 to 5 percent anticipated.[2] Further data need to be collected nationally to validate the inferences drawn from the sample populations from which the original data were collected. By expanding the sample, more accurate trim points may be established. To facilitate this process, institutions need to collect information on LOS and COS per DRG for their population as well as to share data with other similar hospitals.

Errors in DRG assignments constitute another area institutions need to monitor. The errors that occur appear primarily in the sequencing of diagnoses because of incomplete or conflicting documentation. If a DRG assignment is inaccurate, the reimbursement also will be inaccurate and could prove to be quite a problem. The institution may lose appropriate reimbursement or may find upon review that it owes money for excessive reimbursement received. Adequate, accurate documentation is essential for appropriate DRG assignment as well as to facilitate the outlier appeals process.

The last concern is one that all providers should share: the ethics of cost-based care. They must carefully balance the need to be cost efficient with the humanity of practice. Maintaining this balance between needs and resources is supported through quality assurance programs, accreditation processes, and professional standards of practice. Public education and informed consumerism also are important parts of this process.

Several aspects of this system have the potential for affecting professional nursing practice. As institutions gather data and identify mechanisms for problem solving, so must nursing. Using a proactive approach, nursing can establish its significance in the health care arena and control its future.

POTENTIAL NURSING PROBLEMS AND CONCERNS

Financial constraints brought about by changing reimbursement strategies, decreasing patient days, shorter LOS, increased nursing intensity, and expanding outpatient services pose challenges for the future of the nursing profession. Nursing traditionally was viewed as the patient's "mother-surrogate." That image is changing to that of a proactive profit-generating profession that offers the patient (consumer) a unique and highly marketable compendium of skills that can be incorporated into the total package of attaining and maintaining wellness.[3]

Today's nurse is able to utilize these skills to assist patients, family, community, and other health professionals in realistic goal setting and success-oriented, fiscally responsible health care. It is the need for these skills that most frequently necessitates a patient's hospitalization and thus makes nursing an extremely significant profit-generating service. It is nursing's responsibility to facilitate this awareness within the health care arena and to gain autonomy appropriate to its importance. This process will necessitate clearer delineation of accountability for practice as well as the product delivered.

To attain appropriate recognition and gain autonomous accountability, nursing will need to be involved actively in the changes occurring in health care. It must identify the potential impact of these changes on nursing, specifically the PPS, then respond appropriately. To accomplish this, it is necessary first to identify and define the components of professional nursing practice.

MODEL OF PROFESSIONAL NURSING

Professional nursing is a living process that, when effective, reflects a state of balance between the human needs of its clients and the institutional needs of the health care delivery system involved. It is the fluid, continuous link that facilitates the existence of this dyad and allows for the mutual gain attainable in a symbiotic relationship. The practice of professional nursing allows for identification and articulation of human needs through the nursing process. The management of professional nursing practice provides an environment conducive to meeting human needs while attaining institutional goals.

It is essential that practice and management collaborate in an open, trusting, and collegial manner to identify needs, solve problems, and plan for the mutual good of all involved; otherwise, the system becomes fragmented and inefficient. A framework demonstrating this relationship and identifying the components of professional nursing that thread through a system is illustrated in Figure 10–1. The horizontal bar to the right of each component defines its area of major impact on or within the system.

Once defined, the potential impact of the prospective payment system should be addressed according to each component of professional practice (Table 10–2).

Figure 10–1 Model for Professional Nursing Practice

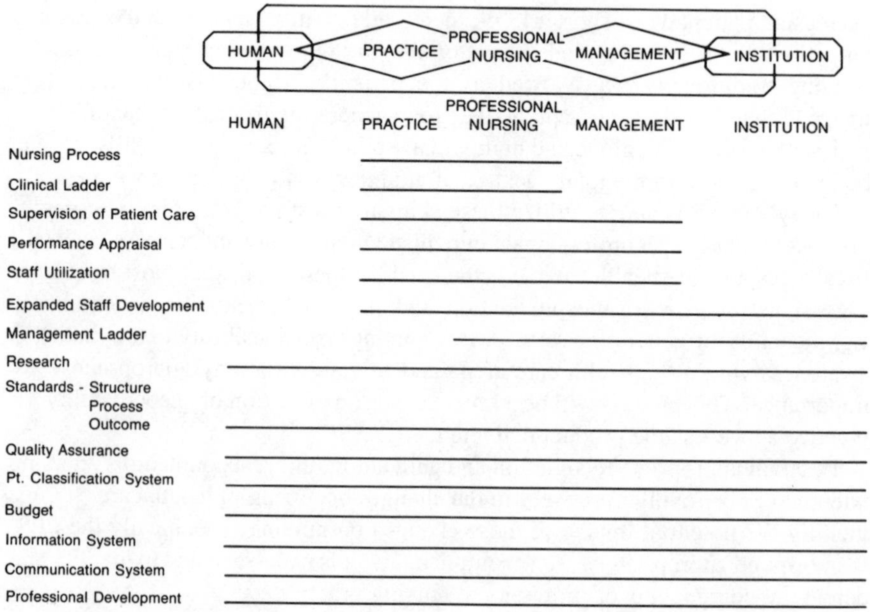

Table 10–2 Potential Constraints to Nursing Under PPS

Components of Nursing Practice	Potential Detrimental Effects
Nursing Process	Value may be decreased because of focus on medical diagnosis and patients' length of stay.
Clinical Ladder	Change in available resources may lead to lack of funds to support various levels of staff that can affect delivery system options. Nursing could become more task oriented if professional practice is not valued.
Management Ladder	Limitation on resources may force consolidation of management positions within nursing. Nursing could lose management control to hospital administration and to M.D.s.
Coordination of Patient Care	Supervision of care may decrease because of limited resources.
Performance Appraisal	Performance could be based on task-oriented medical model, reflecting decreased value for professional practice.
Staff Utilization	Decreasing patient days may be perceived as justification for reduction in nursing care hours when in fact shorter LOS increases intensity of nursing care and need for professional skill mix.
Staff Development	Change in resource base may decrease orientation and continuing education activities; as value for professional nursing practice decreases, need for staff development also drops.
Research	Limitation in resources could make nursing research more difficult.
Standards	Some institutions may lose accreditation while others may choose not to seek it. Nursing as a profession may be threatened by lack of autonomy mandated by standardization from outside nursing.
Quality Assurance	Limited resources may force nursing to respond to cost/benefit or productivity-oriented outcomes, which may not be based on appropriate nursing research.

The utilization of nursing diagnosis as a predictor of patient LOS has the potential of increasing the credibility of the nursing process to those outside the profession.[4] Timely patient and family assessment that facilitates the generation of an appropriate plan of care is imperative. Assessment mechanisms that lead to the identification of nursing diagnoses can and should lend themselves to the development of a plan of care that is patient specific. Interventions that are appropriate to the identified needs of the individual patient should make the best use of resources and demonstrate fiscal responsibility. Coordination of services by a professional nurse who is a dedicated patient advocate will enhance the contribution of nursing to the total program of patient care. Evaluation of care with regard to both quality and financial outcomes is more likely to assure consumers that the best of care is provided for their health care dollars.

Patient/family education must prepare patients to assume responsibility for self-care that once was provided by hospital personnel. Ambulatory care services that facilitate the patients' remaining in their homes or work environments, rather than being hospitalized, must provide relevant information at the consumers' level of understanding. Hospital discharge planning must be designed in a fashion that expedites prompt and safe release, with community support services as needed.

The emphasis on the planning aspect of nursing may suggest that the profession is promoting the role of thinker rather than doer. Ironically, even with the emphasis on the planning and evaluation components of the process, today's nurses must be more highly competent in technical skills than ever. Rapidly advancing technology challenges their ability to assimilate and analyze tremendous amounts of data and to discriminate between the relevant and extraneous information necessary for the delivery of care.

Documentation that satisfies medical-legal and accrediting requirements continues to be the bane of nursing's existence. Some assistance through computerized information systems may help, while contributing to a whole new battery of challenges. As never before, nurses are beginning to correlate specific needs of patients with levels of practice that can best meet those needs.

A career ladder based on the nursing process can increase practitioners' accountability by incorporating specific performance criteria that describe professional expectations. As practitioners ascend either a clinical or management ladder, they should demonstrate increased knowledge and ability to teach and influence others. Clinical experts can have tremendous impact on the economy of patient care by decreasing length of stay, recidivism, and the long-term complications of noncompliance.

Nursing research that facilitates the expansion of assessment methodologies, accurate identification of nursing diagnoses, timely and fiscally accountable nursing interventions, and a comprehensive system of program evaluation will increase the influence and power base of nursing in the health care system.

Identifying the potential constraints of the PPS is the first step in a proactive response for nursing. Table 10–3 identifies one nursing department's example of a plan for increased efficiency and effectiveness during a period of shrinking resources.

The commitment to quality care during a period of constrained resources can pose many challenges to the profession. Nonnursing administrators seeking profit

Table 10–3 Nursing Responses to PPS

Components of Nursing Practice	Appropriate Responses of Nursing

Nursing Process:
  Nursing Diagnosis
  Patient/Family Education
  Discharge Planning
  Technical Skill Competency
  Nursing Research
  Documentation
	Define effects of nursing process on quality of patient outcomes (product).
	Define effects of the cost containment on quality patient outcomes (product).
	Evaluate patient compliance and effect on LOS, recidivism, and subsequent effect on revenues.
	Determine effect on case mix of improved continuity of care, patient education, and discharge planning.

Clinical Ladder	Define practice and increase individual accountability. Evaluate link between level of practice and patient outcome.
Management Ladder	Utilize business skills to improve resource development allocation. Define nursing as a profit center, thereby increasing autonomy, accountability, and value to institution and client.
Coordination of Patient Care	Define need for coordination of patient care by evaluation of LOS, COS, recidivism, and complications.
Performance Appraisal	Evaluate performance based on defined level of practice.
Staff Utilization	Establish skill mix number of nursing staff appropriate to patient case mix and desired patient outcomes. Expect staff utilization to decrease LOS-COS, recidivism, and complications. Interface with schools of nursing to delineate appropriate product.
Staff Development	Increase value and scope of staff development to ensure appropriate orientation and LO practice. Facilitate self-directed professional/personal development.
Nursing Research	Expand theory-based nursing research into clinical practice focus. Investigate and identify most effective and efficient process for attaining desired outcomes. Evaluate relationships among patient acuity, nursing care requirements, and nursing interventions for a specified DRG.
Standards	Assure minimum level of safe, appropriate care for all patients through accountability for clearly defined standards. Identify strategic planning component in nursing for institutional and community needs. Define professional nursing standards in product-oriented terms. Utilize professional nursing research findings to develop and define standards and federal legislation and regulations.
Quality Assurance	Use these activities to define and measure effectiveness and efficiency of nursing care on patient level. Maximize resource utilization to facilitate productivity-focused marketable outcomes at defined level of quality.

and productivity-oriented outcomes may negate the role of the professional nursing staff and opt for service alternatives that appear less costly. The impact of professional nursing practice and a theory base that will support and define the benefits of that practice must be expressed in financial terms. The effect of decreasing lengths of stay in inpatient facilities and reducing unnecessary recidivism and complications because of inadequate patient education and counseling are two examples of ways that nursing might demonstrate its contribution.

Hospitals that once sought the seal of approval given by optional accrediting bodies may be forced to compromise their standards of quality and either not seek accreditation or seek less costly alternatives that will compromise desirable patient outcomes. Unfair competition for patients' health care dollars may arise from the increase in HMOs, surgicenters, and convenience clinics that do not have to meet the accreditation requirements of other facilities. Inadequate input from nursing leaders into hospital and community planning issues may further fragment the delivery of care and decrease appreciation for the holistic approach to wellness.

NURSING INFORMATION SYSTEM

A computerized information system for nursing must address not only the amount of resources required but also the mix, the quality of patient care, individual nurse capabilities, planning and policy-making needs, evaluation, and research. Traditional patient classification schemes group patients according to their physical and emotional needs, observational requirements, and teaching. What is needed in the PPS-DRG era is an automated nursing information system (NIS) comprised of a data base of conditions treated by nurses and interventions provided for those conditions. This data base would facilitate the delineation of nursing's contribution to patient care from admission to discharge.

A NIS identifies nursing's services for both the profession and the consumer. Nursing then becomes accountable for its product at all levels: to the consumer, to the institution, and to the profession. Accountability for a defined level of care enhances nursing's decision-making authority for staffing and budgetary requirements. In addition, NIS provides a computerized data base for long-range planning, quality assurance activities, research, and conversion to a profit-generating department.

In the 1960s, two types of systems for classifying patients according to their nursing care requirements appeared: the prototype and the factor evaluation. Although the latter was considered less subjective and more reliable, both systems were based on nursing tasks performed.[5] By the 1970s, acuity-based staffing was a requirement for accreditation by the Joint Commission on the Accreditation of Hospitals. Sophisticated systems for calculating direct care versus indirect care requirements were described.[6] Yet these systems lacked an overall framework that captured the essence of professional nursing, was applicable to a variety of specialties and health care settings, and differentiated nursing's product from that of other care providers.

The nursing process appeared in the literature for years without a standard diagnostic terminology reflecting in part the evolution of the profession. The inability to consistently label problems that nurses have the knowledge, skill, and experience to treat has hampered the clear delineation of their contribution to health care. However, with the development of nursing diagnosis nomenclature, the product of more than a decade of work by the North American Nursing Diagnosis Association,[7] nursing now has a framework within which to define professional care, applicable to all its specialties across a variety of settings.

Most computerized information systems in the health care industry are based on a medical model, and thus do not address the sophisticated needs of nursing. Nurses involved in data management have a unique opportunity to merge their knowledge of nursing process, utilizing the diagnosis framework and their knowledge of automated information systems, to guide software developers in meeting their special needs.

MODEL NURSING INFORMATION SYSTEM

The impetus for the development of a computerized information system at one midwestern public general teaching hospital arose from the escalating and complex needs stimulated in part by the change to a prospective reimbursement system. That required nursing administrators to have data on the amount and mix of resources needed as well as to match professional nurses' capabilities with individual patient needs to decrease the length and cost of hospitalization without sacrificing the quality of care. The Medicare case mix was important but so, too, was the nursing case mix.

An efficient method of measuring structure, process, and outcome standards became even more important as nursing administrators struggled to control costs under the new budgetary constraints. The importance of a research base to study the links between patient outcomes and nursing interventions was paramount, with increased emphasis on efficiency. It became imperative for hospital administrators to have a mechanism with which to study the patient characteristics of outliers, requiring the merging of nursing, medical, medical record, and financial information systems. With these and many other previously unsolicited information needs becoming apparent, a NIS became imperative.

Considering the numerous times throughout a day a staff nurse would interact with a system, ease of operation or user friendliness was mandatory in designing the model for a nursing information system (Figure 10–2). Nursing interface with the system at the unit level follows the steps of the nursing process.

Figure 10–2 Nursing Information System

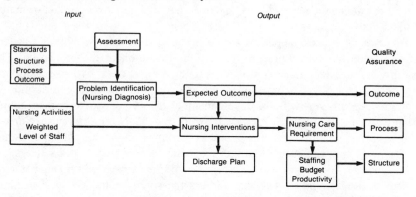

Entering the patient's assessment data is the nurse's initial interaction with the computerized system. The nursing diagnosis framework is used to identify the patient's problems. Process and outcome patient care standards for each nursing diagnosis are preprogrammed as defined by the department. Collaborating with the patient, the nurse selects the appropriate goals and interventions from the preprogrammed menu. When individualized goals or interventions are required, the nurse enters those. The patient's care plan and discharge plan then are printed out as a reference. Revised copies of the plans can be obtained easily when changes are made.

In addition, an acuity assignment (nursing care requirement) is made for the patient based on the preprogrammed weighted nursing interventions chosen from the process standard for each nursing diagnosis. During the patient's hospitalization, nurses enter appropriate documentation in the formatted flow sheets and nurses' notes. At any point during the hospitalization or after discharge, an evaluation of the nursing care and of the patient's progress toward the desired goals can be obtained by comparing what has been documented with the selected goals and interventions and the outcome standards.

The nursing manager can receive the care requirement for each unit, which is a compilation of each patient's nursing intensity. Projected care requirements also can be obtained at any point, since the acuity system is based on the nursing process, and a patient's progress toward an expected outcome can be measured at any time during hospitalization. Productivity reports can be generated by comparing the nursing care requirement of a unit with the actual service delivered. Trends in such requirement can be used to plan long-range staffing and to project budgetary needs. Quality assurance activities are facilitated with a computerized NIS since structure, process, and outcome standards can be compared with documented nursing practice.

BENEFITS OF A NURSING INFORMATION SYSTEM

The data base resulting from a computerized NIS has vast potential for the nursing department from which it is generated as well as for the institution and the profession as a whole. With the aid of an information system a health care facility can define a major component of its product—patient care. The NIS data base facilitates decision making and aids in the strategic planning used in marketing nursing. In addition, the research potential with the aid of a computerized NIS is almost limitless.

Benefits for Nursing

A computerized NIS, using nursing diagnosis as a framework for a patient classification system, provides the basis for a uniform and accurate measure of patients' care requirements across all nursing specialties. Weighted nursing interventions, determined after study to be highly valid and reliable, are based on standards of practice for each specialty area in a facility. The weighted activities for each area include the common physician-ordered interventions as well as nursing orders.

Because this measurement of nursing workload incorporates professional activities in addition to tasks performed under the direction and supervision of a registered nurse, it can be used in any organization where professional nursing is a component. The major advantage of a computerized nursing workload index or patient classification system structured around nursing diagnosis is the ability for nursing to define its practice in virtually any setting.

Once nursing practice in a particular setting is defined, nursing must be accountable for the described level of practice:

- Individual nurses are responsible for providing patients with that defined level of care.
- The nursing department is responsible for providing an environment in which nurses can deliver such care.
- Nursing administrators are responsible for communicating with administrators and physicians to determine that the level of care outlined is appropriate for the facility in the community it serves.

Health care administrators and physicians must have a working knowledge of the services provided by each nursing specialty and use them appropriately. Nurse specialists and administrators must communicate effectively to consumers as to services available and ensure that the defined level of care is provided.

A computerized NIS incorporating a patient classification system based on the nursing process provides the capability for automated quality assurance. Since the weighted activities of that system are based on nursing standards of care, structure, process, and outcome, the quality of care provided can be measured at virtually any time during a patient's hospitalization against the care that should have been provided. At discharge, the desired goal attainment can be measured against what was achieved. Information on any topic on which nursing should want to conduct a quality assurance study would be available on the computerized NIS.

The automated NIS provides a data base to facilitate long-term and short-term decision making. Day-to-day decision making on staffing is facilitated with a workload index that measures nursing's product uniformly across all specialties. Predictive staffing requirements are possible since the system is based on the nursing process, and a patient's progress toward goal attainment can be ascertained at any time. Productivity studies are facilitated and can be matched with trends in nursing case mix for long-term planning purposes. Budget justification for staffing is enhanced. Because nursing's product is uniform across specialties, the costing of its services is facilitated, thereby creating the possibility of transforming it into a profit-generating department.

The NIS also offers a data base for nursing research. Reasons for the paucity of research on nursing practice issues included the lack of a standard terminology and lack of access to a data base.[8] Care delivery systems can be studied for their efficiency in meeting predetermined outcomes. Nursing intervention and outcome links can be studied for any number of patient problems. Patient adherence with prescribed plans can be studied to identify effective teaching methodologies. Certain patient characteristics (e.g., sensory/perceptual deficits, lack of support systems) can be linked with increased length-of-stay and recidivism rates.

The educational level and experience of nursing staff can be examined in relation to the efficiency and effectiveness with which patient outcomes are reached. The intensity of nursing care within and across DRGs—that is, nursing case mix—can be determined. Nursing intervention can be studied in relation to length of stay, cost of hospitalization, and recidivism rates.

Benefits for the Health Care Facility

In addition to a data base for nursing, a computerized NIS also provides the health care facility with a new dimension for its own data base. Program planning for the institution is enhanced, systemwide problems are identified more easily, program planning needs for the community can be pinpointed, and the facility's research base gains an invaluable new dimension.

The addition of nursing information to the hospital's data base provides an opportunity for studying case-mix details. Linked with other information systems in the facility (i.e., medical records, financial), NIS helps identify program planning needs.

For example, before NIS, it may have been known that the length of stay for patients over age 70 usually exceeded the Medicare maximum. With the addition of the nursing information to the data base, an administrator now may discern that this group of patients also experienced impaired mobility and lack of support systems in the home. With this additional information, a program can be planned to deal with these problems on admission to facilitate earlier discharges.

The NIS offers an enhanced ability to identify systemwide problems. As with the previous example, awareness of a problem may exist but the specific cause may remain elusive without nursing data. For example, the recidivism rate for patients with a particular diagnosis—urinary diversion—may be unusually high. The addition of data from the NIS may provide insight into possible causes: knowledge deficit, self-care deficit, infection, or skin integrity problems.

The NIS makes available to the health care facility information in a newer and perhaps faster form for input into program planning for the community. Again, the example of extended length of stay for a population over 70 is appropriate. NIS data may demonstrate that patients were ready for discharge to a skilled nursing facility on the designated date. Further exploration may indicate, however, that the availability of skilled nursing beds in the community is limited, forcing an extension of the length of stay for patients requiring those services. The NIS data may indicate that these patients could be discharged several days earlier if an environment of supervised living were available in the community. The health care facility can use such data to provide community leaders with information needed for future planning.

Perhaps the most important advantage of an NIS for a health care facility is the research data base it provides. Factors in addition to case mix can be correlated with extended length of stay, high-cost hospitalizations, and outliers. This can be compared with information from similar health care facilities to form a regional data base. This information could even have an impact nationally on reimbursement rates, exclusions (e.g., public general hospitals), and priorities for health care funding.

A computerized NIS incorporating a patient classification system founded in the nursing process thus can have a substantial impact on nursing and on a health care institution. The system requires nursing to define its services in a uniform fashion, applicable to all its specialties in a variety of settings. This can enable nursing to become a profit center accountable for the quality of the product it provides, and responsible for the cost of its services and revenue generated. A computerized information system for nursing also can enhance strategic planning and policy-making decisions by nursing and by the facility by providing an expanded, accessible research data base.

NOTES

1. P.L. Grimaldi and J.A. Micheletti, *Diagnosis Related Groups: A Practitioner's Guide* (Chicago: Pluribus Press, 1983), p. 5.

2. P.L. Grimaldi and J.A. Micheletti, *Diagnosis Related Groups: A Practitioner's Guide* (Chicago: Pluribus Press, 1983), p. 217.

3. W.J. Riley and V. Schaefers, "Nursing Operations as a Profit Center," *Nursing Management* 15, no. 4 (April, 1984), 43–46.

4. R.M. Toth, "Reimbursement Mechanism Based on Nursing Diagnosis," in *Classification of Nursing Diagnoses: Proceedings of the Fifth National Conference*, ed. M.J. Kim, G.K. McFarland and A.M. McLean (St. Louis: The C.V. Mosby Company, 1984), pp. 90–102.

5. P. Giovannetti, "Understanding Patient Classification Systems," *Journal of Nursing Administration* 4, no. 9 (February 1979), 4–9.

6. C.N. Tomsky, "Acuity-Based Staffing Controls Costs," *Nursing Management* 14, no. 10 (October, 1983), 36–37.

7. M.J. Kim, G.K. McFarland, and A.M. McLean, *Classification of Nursing Diagnoses* (St. Louis: The C.V. Mosby Company, 1984), p. ix.

8. Study Group on Nursing Information Systems, "Computerized Nursing Information Systems: An Urgent Need," *Research in Nursing and Health* 6, no. 3 (September, 1983), 101–105.

Index

Index